The Girlfriend EXperience

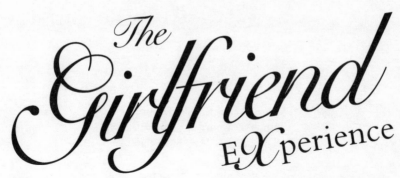

The Girlfriend EXperience

My fun and adventurous life as an escort

Rebecca 'Bea' Dakin

JOHN BLAKE

Published by John Blake Publishing Ltd,
3 Bramber Court, 2 Bramber Road,
London W14 9PB, England

www.johnblakepublishing.co.uk

First published in paperback in 2009

ISBN: 978-1-84454-752-4

British Library Cataloguing-in-Publication Data:

A catalogue record for this book is available from the British Library.

Design by www.envydesign.co.uk

Printed in the UK by CPI William Clowes Beccles NR34 7TL

1 3 5 7 9 10 8 6 4 2

Papers used by John Blake Publishing are natural, recyclable
products made from wood grown in sustainable forests.
The manufacturing processes conform to the environmental r
egulations of the country of origin.

Every attempt has been made to contact the relevant copyright-holders,
but some were unobtainable. We would be grateful if the appropriate
people could contact us.

I dedicate this book to a few people. Firstly my Grandma Edith: I miss you every day. Secondly to Mum and Dad for your unconditional love, and lastly to all my other family and friends who never judged me and who accept me for who I am.

The art of peace emanated from the Divine Form and the Divine Heart of existence; it reflects the true, good, beautiful, and absolute nature of creation and the essence of its ultimate grand design. The purpose of the Art of Peace is to fashion sincere human beings; sincere human being is one who has unified body and spirit, one who is free of hesitation or doubt, and one who understands the power of words.

The totally awakened warrior can freely utilize all elements contained in heaven and earth. The true warrior learns how to correctly perceive the activity of the universe and how to transform martial techniques into vehicles of purity, goodness and beauty. A warrior's mind and body must be permeated with enlightened wisdom and deep calm.

Morihei Ueshiba (1883–1969)
From *The Art Of Peace: Quotes from Morihei Ueshiba* translated and edited by John Stevens.

Disclaimer:
Various names, places, details and situations have been changed for legal reasons.

Acknowledgements

My thanks to John Blake, for eventually (with some gentle persuasion and my persistence) believing in me, my book and my ability as a writer. You were right; I could do it on my own!

Also thanks to my editors at Blake – Dan for initially reading my blurb and helping me format chapters and put it in some sort of order, and Vicky for her invaluable advice on the reformatting of my book. All your changes were for the better! And lastly to Allie, thank you for helping me in these crucial final stages.

I was initially inspired to write my story after reading the anonymous *Belle De Jour*. I was compelled to write my story and show a very different side of escorting – the less seedy side, and the social side of escorting. So thank you Belle (if you exist!) for inspiring me.

I should also thank all my clients over the years, for giving me so many wonderful experiences and opportunities that otherwise I'd never have had. I can't thank you enough. Those of you who I've written about, I hope you think I have been discreet enough – thank you for giving me the material and inspiration to write. To my regulars that have stuck by me for years – T, G, J and J, a special thank you and lots of love to you.

To my friends and family who have contributed to my book with your thoughts on me and my profession, huge thanks. I know we've all got busy lives so it really is appreciated that you took the time to write your thoughts for me – Sensei, Pete, Keith, Katie G, Aunty Sue, Vickie, JZ, Daniel James, Andy, Andrea, Aunty Kate, Jenny, Nat and last but by no means least Mum. You have all played an essential part in the balance of my book. I can't thank you enough.

Aunty Kate – thanks for reading through all my literature and advising me. You've been an absolute star!

Nat – You've known me half my life. Thanks for reading my earlier attempts at writing, your input in the book, and also for passing various extracts around your office for feedback. You've encouraged and believed in me all the years I've been writing – a massive thank you to you.

Paola – Many thanks for reading through and advising me on how to tweak a few of my diary entries.

Sensei Ken – My life has changed for the better since I joined your dojo and you introduced me to the art of Aikido. As the years go by I can feel my confidence building and I am growing both spiritually and mentally – many thanks to you and to all your staff at the dojo for all your emotional support, encouragement and for believing in me and helping me believe in my self.

To all my family and friends, thank you for your patience over the past five years as I changed from a social butterfly to a writer and consequently a hermit, and for understanding and accepting my lack of calls, and time to meet.

I've had a few rocks over the past few years. Keith – my very dear friend, thank you for consistently being there, listening and supporting me. Another special thank you to my dear

ACKNOWLEDGEMENTS

gentleman friend T, you know who you are. I don't know what I would have done without you over these past few years! You're my guardian angel. R, you've been a very supportive friend, over my years as an escort as you have advised me on the forums, my photos and website and patiently guided me through many problems with my total lack of computer knowledge (I know I haven't got any better, but I've got other skills!) Last but by no means least, my gorgeous friend S, who's supported me in the biz. I can't imagine working all these years as an escort without you as a friend. Thank you!

Big thanks again to Mick, my web designer @ MGF who has also put up with my ignorance about computers and has offered consistent support and advice well above the call of duty, on a number of occasions. You've been very good to me. Thank you!

A number of biographies and autobiographies by people I admire also inspired me during my time writing, so my thanks also to Sharon Osbourne, Richard Branson, Tina Turner, Simon Cowell, Katie Price, Gordon Ramsay, Madonna and Paul O'Grady.

During my early writing days I was fortunate enough to exchange emails with the author of one of my favourite books, *The Game* by Neil Strauss. I initially contacted him thinking I might be able to help with a book he was writing. This never happened but he did write some encouraging words to me about writing my book, so my thanks to you Neil. I hope you'll read and enjoy my book as much as I did yours.

And finally thank you to my parents for 'putting up' with me, even whilst I tested the boundaries of unconditional love. I love you both dearly!

Contents

Introduction

So, what's Andrew doing now?' asked Jane, the family friend my mother hadn't seen for years. 'He's working as a tree surgeon for one of his friends, and Peter is in telecommunications,' she said of my two brothers, aged 28 and 30. My sister Sarah, 26 at the time, explained that she was working in Trading Standards for the council. 'And what about Rebecca?' Jane's husband Paul asked. 'She now works as a high-class escort,' said Mum, with as much normality as she could muster. 'So she's a hooker?' Paul countered triumphantly, with a big grin. Embarrassed, my Mum then tried to explain that I wasn't a hooker and that I travelled all over the world, going to prestigious hotels and restaurants with businessmen.

Like most people, I used to think escorts/call girls/prostitutes/whores/hookers were all the same, but now I don't. I have nothing against prostitution or anyone in the sex trade, but the only word I would use for my profession is 'escort'. The reason for this is that I sell my time: sex is not guaranteed, it is always my choice. I specialise in offering a 'GFE' – what's known in the business as 'the Girlfriend Experience' – which I guess translates as a 'hired girlfriend'. In other words, I spend long periods of time with the guys who choose to see me and we both take time to get to know one another. Most of my dates are overnights and dinner dates, but I also go away for short breaks. A very small percentage of my time is spent entertaining in the bedroom; most of my time on a date is taken up with socialising and dining.

It's a common misconception that men only pay escorts for sex. Men are a lot more in need of affection and companionship, and the feeling that they are attractive, listened to and wanted, than we women give them credit for.

Some escorts would consider themselves prostitutes and some blatantly advertise their sexual services. Some people think there is no difference. Everyone interprets things differently. After you've read my book, why not make up your own mind?

Diary: February 2008

I haven't seen John since last year. I only get to see him when his wife's away, which isn't often enough.

John was looking for affection after his wife moved into a spare room, saying he snored. When they did share a bed he was never allowed to cuddle her and a couple of years ago she decided she wanted to move into the spare room. This is when he started searching for an escort. Apparently she only goes into his room when she wants sex. He never knows if it will happen or not, so he sits in his room waiting to see if he gets called on. The vision of this does make me chuckle; it sounds very clinical. She sounds stricter than me! He's a really lovely guy, and it's sad he doesn't get the affection he needs from his wife.

John is 75, but looks much younger. He's over six feet tall, very fit and strong, and keeps himself trim. He has a full head of unruly grey hair. What I love about him is his great sense of humour, which is very dry, sarcastic and cheeky, much like mine. He's extremely wealthy and generous, and usually takes me shopping when we meet to buy me expensive clothes and jewellery.

I really look forward to seeing him because I am genuinely very fond of him. I'm very comfortable and relaxed around him so we both enjoy our meetings. I have found that the older guys are generally more chilled.

My booking was for an extended overnight date that was to start at 6p.m. and finish at midday the next day. I've met him around twelve times, so we are very comfortable around each other, and I was looking forward to seeing him. He lives in Scotland, but flies down to meet me a couple of times a year.

I had booked us a table at a local restaurant for dinner that evening. When I arrived at the hotel, I gave him a massive hug and the bag of gifts I had bought him for Christmas.

I had found him a new leather glasses case (his old one was dog-eared) and a leather tidy tray for his bedroom for his keys and coins. He always says I shouldn't buy him presents, but I love buying him things because he's so generous to me and his family, and he never buys anything for himself.

Apologising, he said that he didn't think he'd be able to take me shopping this time because his cat was ill and he was going to have to leave early. 'Damn that cat!' I thought. I told him that I hadn't expected it (although I'd secretly hoped) and that I totally understood. After an hour of chat we wandered over to the restaurant.

The owner smiled and winked at me as I walked through the restaurant door first. I'm sure he knows I'm an escort after seeing me with numerous older men. He greeted us warmly, while taking our jackets and directing us to the lounge.

We both ordered non-alcoholic cocktails as we perused the menu. A teenage couple looked at us curiously as we began our banter, laughing at each other's cheeky comments.

They always bring intricate canapés that look too good to eat before we begin our meal. Whenever I can't choose between two dishes from the menu, John will always tell me to order both, and when I say I won't be able to eat it all, he insists it doesn't matter. I know he's serious, but I'd never do it. My mum brought me up not to be greedy and to eat everything on my plate! Even now I feel guilty and I'm apologetic if I can't finish my food on my dates.

John has a very sweet tooth and couldn't decide which of the desserts to have, so he ordered all five. 'Sir, we do an assiette of desserts, which is five smaller portions – a little of everything on the dessert menu,' he was informed. Our waitress kept trying to explain how big the portions were; she wouldn't listen to him. But he knew how big the desserts were, and he wanted five. Eventually she got the message and they came out, one by one. He finished every single mouthful. God knows where he puts it all!

I always tell him off for pestering the waitresses. He jumps the gun: he's even more impatient than me and that's saying something! For example, when we've finished our mains, he'll ask for the dessert menu without giving them a chance to offer it, then when we've finished, he'll request the bill again without allowing them a moment to ask if he wants it. Then when we get the bill, he asks for his coat without giving them a chance to offer it. So I'll tease him and tell him to behave, and not be so impatient. He just laughs and tells me I'm lovely.

After a leisurely dinner, he requested the bill. They add a service charge, but he always tips them heavily on top of that, and when the young girl came with the card machine she told him the service charge was included. He knew it was and said it was OK. I don't know how much extra he had put on, but the look of shock on the girl's face was enough. 'Are you sure?' she asked, looking extremely unsure herself. He told her it was fine. 'Oh, thank you, thank you so much, that's very kind of you, thank you...' she rambled, bowing gratefully and then scurrying off.

Back at the room we dimmed the lights and lit candles. We put on some music (Newton Faulkner, for some relaxing acoustic guitar) and I stood on tiptoes to kiss him; we swayed to the music, embracing each other.

We fumbled about removing our clothes before lying down to get more comfortable. He loves to give me oral sex so he soon moved between my legs, gently parting them so he could lie between them. He's very good at giving me oral sex, but I never climax, probably because he's always asking me why I don't, so I feel under pressure and never relax fully enough for it to happen.

After pleasuring me he moved up my body, kissing up my torso, stopping momentarily at my breasts before moving back up to my lips. He loves his nipples to be pinched and sucked really hard (he's only found that out since he's been with me as we've experimented together). So I reached to pinch his nipple and his breathing got shorter and more frantic as he groaned in pleasure. He doesn't always want me to give him oral sex, and this time he didn't so he played with my breasts and I pinched and sucked his nipples as he grew more and more excited.

I've never made him come yet, as he hasn't with me, but I never mention it because I know I don't like it when he questions why he can't make me climax. He climaxes with his wife, so it's a bit disheartening that I can't make him because I know he wants to. I believe she tries harder than me and is far more patient. They probably make love for hours, whereas foreplay and fun lasts only about an hour or so with me.

I'd ordered breakfast for 8.30a.m. It always feels very decadent to eat breakfast in bed. I love it! I woke when it arrived and we ate in bed... boiled eggs and soldiers, you can't beat it! Then I left, leaving him to shower and check on his cat. He still paid me for the extended date.

When I got home and counted my envelope, he'd given me £1,200. A few days later he sent me a gift of £1,500 – I think because he felt guilty he hadn't taken me shopping.

CHAPTER 1:

The Black Sheep

I consider my parents and family 'normal', whatever that means. I come from a stable, close family and no one else has chosen such a risqué profession.

My family is working-class. I am the eldest and the most responsible, in some respects (I'm sure they would disagree), of four. Although the relationship with my family is now getting stronger, I still consider myself to be the Black Sheep. It used to upset me that I was different, but now I am happy and content with the person I am.

My dad is an only child and he met my mum when she was teaching in his hometown in Derbyshire. He was a navigator in the Merchant Navy and my mum was lucky enough to be able to travel the world with him. Mum is from a large farming family in Dorset and she carried on their tradition by having four of us. After Dad left the Navy, he took over the family newsagent business in Matlock. It was a thriving business, but newspapers and magazines only make a small profit, so as a family we weren't considered well off. My parents chose to spend any spare money they had on our education, sending us all to a private primary school. They still live in the house they bought years ago, but Dad added an extension so we could all have our own rooms.

We didn't have holidays abroad, but we always had fun, even if we were all in a tent on my granny's farm for our summer holidays! My mum was a very 'hands on' mum and used to take all of us and our friends for picnics and to beautiful countryside spots. One of our favourites was Robin Hood Stride, which was a bunch of rocks to climb. We'd take a picnic and there would be eight of us (because if one of us had a friend coming along, we all wanted to invite someone) and my mum, rammed like sardines in her big old rusty red Marina.

At primary school we were very much the odd ones out, as nearly everyone came from rich families. I dreaded 'Own Clothes Day', when I would have to rummage through bin bags of second-hand clothes passed down from my mum's good friend's daughter, Helen. I hated most of them, but there'd be the odd wearable thing. None of it was fashionable so I wouldn't say they were gratefully received by me. Struggling to clothe four children, my mum was always thankful for them, though.

I do remember being very sexually aware from an early age. I was fascinated with boobs and when I went to Helen's I used to suggest that we go round to her neighbour's and pinch Page 3 from his newspaper. It used to excite me, looking at the boobs. I've since found out that Helen is a lesbian.

I would also fantasise about my parents' friends in an inappropriate way. I don't know where this came from – Mum and Dad are not openly affectionate and I never caught them in any compromising positions. We weren't even allowed to watch anything unsuitable on TV and my parents were very strict about the ratings on films. Dad didn't even sell top-shelf magazines in his newsagent's, and neither of them spoke to any of us kids about sex.

I recall teaching numerous friends how to masturbate; of course at the time I didn't realise what I was doing. When Mum put our socks into pairs she would tuck one into the other and this would make a long sausage shape. I'd put it down my trousers, or up my skirt, and lie on my front and then writhe about. I just knew it made me warm and tingly down below, so I told friends and showed them how to do it. I'd meaningfully snog a pillow too, and fantasise about being with a man, usually Shakin' Stevens behind the Green Door! I'm not sure what prompted me to do this, as I know I was the opposite of my well-behaved sister as she was growing up – she never did anything similar.

Once I was told off and sent home for teaching one of my parents' friends' daughters how to play husband and wife. I was maybe 11 or so, and she was a few years younger than me. Her parents came in and she was writhing about on her top bunk, pretending to be with a man. We were simulating sex, but at the time I didn't know what sex actually involved.

Although I was very sexually aware, I was insecure about my looks and I believe this stems from being made to have short hair as a child. It was only about two inches long all over, so no boys ever fancied me. Often I would be asked if I was a boy or a girl and I hated this, as I'm sure you can imagine. When I was still in primary school I remember saying that I was going to have plastic surgery on my face when I grew up. Even though I now know that I was a pretty child, my short hair made me feel ugly. Being so young, I thought that plastic surgery involved having my face bandaged up for a few weeks, and then when the bandages were removed, I would be beautiful. If I'd known they actually cut you open, I wouldn't have said that! I used to have a recurring dream that I was looking in the mirror; I had long hair and I was beautiful. I constantly told my mum I hated myself and was ugly. Unfortunately, she never took these comments seriously.

I was a handful for my parents as a child. Because of my

insecurities I constantly wanted attention and reassurance. I am embarrassed to say that I used to feel very hard done by because I suffered with hay fever (which was extremely inconvenient when we spent time on the farms as I often missed out on fun with my siblings during the hay making season) and various allergies. I often had bloody patches on my skin, where I had scratched my eczema, and I have also had various problems with arthritis throughout my life. All my siblings seemed to be perfect – everything I wasn't. They didn't suffer from any of the conditions I had, and in my eyes they were all attractive and I was the ugly one. Being the eldest I got the blame for everything my siblings did, whether I was with them or not, and if I fell out with friends at school, Mum would always ask what I'd done to them. Everything seemed to be my fault and this contributed to my lack of confidence. My school reports consistently said I lacked confidence in my ability, and people still tell me this now, so writing this book has been a big positive step. My dad was always considered the soft touch in our family and my mum was the disciplinarian, an old-fashioned one too. I didn't feel like my parents cared about how I felt because I was never taken seriously – I still feel this to a certain extent even now.

I had various ideas of what I wanted to be when I grew up. Had I known such a thing as stage school existed and that maybe I could become a singer or an actress, I believe I would have found my vocation. As a young child I thought that famous singers were just born that way; I wasn't aware that I could have been anything I wanted to be. I wouldn't say I was particularly good at singing or acting, but being a natural show-off and entertainer, I believe I could have worked at it and it would have fed me the attention I craved. As far as acting went, I was never given a chance to shine as I was always put in the chorus, both at school and in the local drama group.

I have an early memory of having friends round and miming to Madonna with a hairbrush (like so many of us did), but then I'd get my friends to sit on the floor and pretend to be my fans, shouting, 'I love you!' and screaming, trying to grab me. OK, I know it sounds very weird, but looking back it was clear I wanted to entertain and also to be admired.

As I didn't believe it was possible to be a singer, I would always say I wanted to be a fashion designer. My mum said I was always very conscious of fashion and beauty from a very early age. I'm not sure why, when as a family we couldn't afford new clothes and my mum wasn't at all like that.

By the time I got to secondary school I was allowed to grow my hair into a bowl cut, which accentuated my round, fat face. This was the start of the verbal bullying I suffered, which carried on for years. I was made to think that my round face was ugly; I know now that it isn't, but I am still self-conscious. I would cry at the hairdresser's and tell my mum how much I hated it, how ugly I was, but she wouldn't listen to me; she just kept telling me I was beautiful.

For years, I was bullied by the boys at school in Chesterfield and in Matlock to the point where I considered myself so repulsive that I thought I would never, ever have a boyfriend. I never told anyone about the bullying, I just accepted it because I didn't think anyone would do anything, and I'm ashamed to say my friend and I actually verbally bullied other girls because to me it seemed to be the norm.

Despite this, I was well liked by the girls at school and loved to make people laugh, so I became a bit of an entertainer. I did this ridiculous impression of a chicken (I have no idea how it came about or what my inspiration was). About fifteen girls would all be sitting on the school field, asking me to lay an egg on them! I would walk in between them all and randomly pick girls to 'lay an egg' on. Then I would squawk and do these funny faces and a silly walk; people would howl with laughter.

The bullying at school, with lads calling me 'Football Face' among other things, made me feel extremely self-conscious. Out of school I would plaster my face with heavy make-up. It took me about forty minutes to apply it all, and for me it was a mask to hide my hideous face. I would also hide my face in my hands at any opportunity. When I laughed, I put my hand in front of my face because I thought laughing made my face look fatter and rounder. Even now I still feel uncomfortable with my hair up.

I didn't French-kiss anyone until I was 14. At that age I became totally obsessed with my friend's brother, Sheldon, who was 16. He was one of the few guys I had met who didn't bully me and for this reason, I believed him to be very mature. He made me feel normal and not self conscious. I was dreading him ever finding out that I was known as 'Football Face'. I loved his sense of humour – he had me in stitches constantly, and he was the first guy to actually flirt with me. I thought I was in love.

One night I went round to their house and we snuck out and climbed on some hay bales, where we sat for hours, having a laugh and drinking beer. Hoping he would make a move if he thought I was drunk, after a couple of sips I began wobbling and rambling on. It was a poor act and he must have known I was putting it on, but he ended up carrying me back to bed (I remember being really chuffed that my plan worked), and it was a like a dream... I felt like Anne of Green Gables, the ugly duckling ending up with the handsome husband. It was one of my favourite films because I related to her character. It made me feel I had hope of finding love, as Anne was bullied for how she looked and the most popular guy at school who used to bully her ultimately ended up romancing her. I was fantasising about spending the rest of my life with Sheldon and I hadn't even kissed him!

After a few months of flirting, we took the next step. One day, we were playing hide and seek; Sheldon and I were hiding in the same spot outside, under some ferns. As we were lying down, he commented that he could see my pink knickers! For some reason I thought this was a compliment and I began to blush (my face and down below). I remember it clearly: there we were among the ferns, me blushing and feeling all tingly, and he started to kiss me. I was terrified that I'd do something wrong, but I was so excited that finally someone thought I was attractive enough to kiss! Next thing I knew, my friend shouted that she could see us. Damn her! Luckily she didn't see what we were up to.

The next time I saw my best friend at school, I excitedly recalled every detail. Each time I saw Sheldon after that I'd get so excited, thinking it might go further. I was crazy about him, and he and his whole family knew. I was *so* obvious! I kissed him one more time after that amazing moment, and then my world fell apart.

I was getting on the bus back to Matlock one day, with my best friend Katie, and Sheldon was at the back. As usual, I blushed at the sight of him, especially as I was wearing my school uniform. Then, as I sat down, I heard the usual chants of 'Football Face'. To my horror, Sheldon started chanting along with them. My best friend asked, with a smirk, 'Isn't Sheldon shouting "Football Face"?' I was mortified.

My friend Katie and I loved *Twin Peaks* when we were 13 or 14, and followed the American cult TV series obsessively. One episode showed the beautiful Sherilyn Fenn trying to get a job at a brothel. She was given the once-over: a quick look up and down by the Madam, before being told there weren't any vacancies. On the side of the Madam's desk was a bowl of cherries. Sherilyn plucked one, ate it and removed the stalk from her plump lips tied in a knot; she was given a job there and then. Katie and I immediately went to the supermarket, bought a carton of cherries and spent the afternoon perfecting the trick. A few years ago, I had an escort job visiting a couple and impressed them with this party piece!

Anyhow, I tried to accept that I was never going to have a 'normal' life. I believed that wherever I went, everyone would find out my nickname and I would be stuck with it for the rest of my life. I would never get married or settle down because I was repulsive to men.

I was thrilled when a guy I fancied in Matlock wanted to go out with me. We went out for three months and I lost my virginity to him. I was 15. We planned to have sex one night after a couple of months together, when his mum and dad were out. I remember being in absolute agony as he tried to penetrate me. Of course there was no real foreplay, so I was probably dry as a bone. It's no wonder it hurt like hell! I just remember wanting it to be over as quickly as possible. We did it a few times after that, but it was still really painful for me, so I didn't enjoy it. Just as I'd started to get used to having sex and was actually on my way to discovering how enjoyable it could be, he dumped me for no apparent reason. He said he hated me.

Distraught, I thought I'd never find a boyfriend again. I'd waited 15 years to find one guy, and he'd dumped me. I never found out why. As far as I was aware, there was no one else, so I was left feeling hurt and angry.

I went out with a very good-looking guy called Keith for three months, but I thought he was too attractive, and being insecure I didn't trust him. I remember being really surprised that someone so good-looking fancied me. It fizzled out after a few months because once I left school I spent three years studying in various places. We saw each other occasionally for a few years until I met James, my first real boyfriend. I'm still in touch with Keith now and he's one of my very best friends.

When I was 15 I started sleeping around with older guys because I thought that if people wanted to have sex with me, it meant I was attractive. I was mature for my age and people always assumed I was older than I was. Most guys I met said they found me intriguing – they could never tell how I felt, or what I was thinking. It's for this reason that I believe I didn't fit into the standard teenage mould. I didn't need or expect anything from men and was always in control of my feelings; I never let anyone get close. Something in me switched after the rejection of my first boyfriend and I guess I just put barriers up to avoid being hurt again. If I was in control, seeing lots of guys and never caring for any of them, then I wouldn't get hurt again.

I used to get a buzz out of being this sexual woman – well, girl – who intrigued men. Though I never had an orgasm, I used to love to perform and entertain men. The more I didn't care, the more they seemed to crave my attention. After so much negativity from the opposite sex, I made the most of it.

Although in some ways I was mature, deep down I was young and naïve. I know now that there are many men who will go with anyone, especially a young girl, if they are looking for an easy lay. It did improve my confidence, but it certainly wasn't the best way to do it!

By the time I left school, I knew people were staring all the time and mocking me because of how I looked, so I decided I would really give them something to talk about. Matlock is a very small town, so I used to get a kick out of being different and became an exhibitionist. I loved that people talked about me and knew who I was.

I had a 1960s see-through lace dress that I would wear with a push-up bra and a thong. It doesn't sound all that outrageous now, but at the time it was (unless you were part of the Rock or Fetish scene). I used to go out in Nottingham, Chesterfield and Derby, and people didn't dress like that in the dance clubs or cheesy nightclubs. I wore suspenders and hot pants, and once travelled all the way down to London to buy some clear plastic trousers, which I wore with a silver thong bikini. My favourite was a black rubber dress that was £20 from the Condom Shop in Leeds, and a chain-mail bra. I began to actually get off on all the attention.

At this point, I was hanging around with people much older than me. My mum wanted me to invite them round for tea, but they were all in their twenties, with their own homes, and it just would not have been cool! She couldn't understand because she knew all of my siblings' friends. I was always the least close to my family because I felt that they never really understood me; the times I did invite people of my own age round, Mum would embarrass me by shouting at me for one reason or another, so I had no intention of taking my older friends home.

With them, I went to all-night raves at the weekend, and I started taking drugs. I never got hooked, it was just when I went clubbing – drugs like Ecstasy, amphetamines, cocaine, acid and ketamine were everywhere on the rave scene. I loved going to the clubs because people accepted me and I always got lots of positive attention, especially from men; I felt accepted and normal. Nobody ever bullied me or made fun of me, and I was seen as being sexy. The Ecstasy people took made everyone feel 'loved-up', and people were so friendly. I would wish the week away at school and look forward to the weekend, when I would take my earnings from working at Dad's shop and spend it on getting into a club, usually Shelley's in Stoke or the Warehouse in Doncaster.

At the time, I'd never demand anything emotionally from men. When I was 16, I was seeing a 35-year-old man, which in retrospect is quite disturbing. He worked as an MC in one of the clubs; women threw themselves at him, and I had his phone number. I never threw myself at him and didn't care if he went off with someone else – I was never jealous. I always let him come to me, and he would call me if he wanted to see me; I never called him once. Even girls much older than me were obsessed with him, and called and pestered him all the time. I was seeing other men too, so the attention he got didn't bother me, and because I was so chilled, we stayed friends for about eight years.

I was 17 when one of my older friends suggested he should pimp me out. He showed me contact magazines and said that he could arrange for me to get paid for sex; he said he'd drive me to see these guys and sit outside the room while I went in and had sex for money. He'd take a cut, and knowing him it would probably have been a big one, which is why I didn't want to do it. Because of my promiscuity the idea didn't shock me – I slept with guys I didn't care about anyway, so why not get paid for it? Thankfully, though, I never accepted his offer.

My parents despaired and didn't know what to do for the best. I didn't want to have anything to do with my family; I'd rather go raving than spend a quiet evening at the weekend in the pub with them, mainly because I felt unhappy around them, so it was a constant battle. I had no connection with them whatsoever, which was partly my fault for being 'different' and not fitting in; I wanted to spend time with people who made me feel good about myself – my friends. It wasn't intentional, I'm sure, but my family hindered rather than helped my confidence. My parents knew about the drugs, but I think they were in denial. I'd look awful when I got home from a rave – after dancing non-stop for 17 hours I would literally have lost half a stone in weight. My mum would try to get me to sit down and have Sunday dinner, and I'd just want to go to my room and play rave music. Because of my age, I suppose it must have been difficult for them to spot what was normal unsociable teenage behaviour and what was down to drug use – being the eldest, they didn't really know how to deal with me. Mum tried grounding me, but when I was allowed out again, I'd lie and pretend I'd gone to a friend's when in fact I would go raving. I told my dad that I was going through a 'phase' and that the best thing to do would be to let it run its course. That 'phase' lasted about ten years!

Diary: July 2008

'Can I call you back, Bea? I'm just shooting.'
'Of course, are you clay pigeon shooting?'
'No, I'm shooting real pigeons!'

Sounds like my kinda guy! This was Colin, from Cork, and we met last night for a dinner date in Birmingham. He sounded adorable on the phone; he checked with me to see if 50 was too old for me... Hardly, he's a spring chicken compared to most of the guys I see!

He was over on business and he sounded laidback and fun on the phone. Generally, the Irish guys I see for work are. However, my heart did sink a little when he asked if we could have room service on our dinner date. 'Er... no,' I politely told him, but said that if he was concerned about bumping into his two colleagues, as he suggested, I could meet him at a restaurant in town and we could discreetly go back to the room separately. It seems he wasn't that concerned about bumping into them because he said it would be fine and we'd eat at the hotel, so I think he was just trying it on.

I would be getting a train to Birmingham and then a taxi back, so that I didn't get back too late. He would be dressed casually, so I put on some smart jeans and a low-cut plain V-neck black top with a bit of jewellery.

On the short walk down to the hotel, I called my local cab firm and asked if someone could pick me up from Birmingham.

I waltzed confidently into the modern-looking trendy hotel, going straight past Reception. I didn't know where I was going, but fortunately the lifts were right in front of me. As I jumped in, I realised I needed a key card to operate the lift and I was going to be stuck. For a few seconds, I stood staring at the panel in the lift until a guy got in as the doors were closing and inserted his key card. My date was staying on the top floor, the 17th. I wondered if it would be the Presidential Suite or similar.

The corridors and doors were all wooden, giving the hotel a Scandinavian look. I'd never been to this hotel, but I'd had a nosey on the Web and it looked great, especially the restaurant and spa.

I knocked, but there was no answer. I was pretty sure he'd be there as we'd been in contact throughout the day; he'd even asked if I wanted to call him in his room. I called him and thought it was just about to go to answer-phone when he picked up. He said he was coming down the stairs, so I wasn't sure where he was. Was there a staircase in the room, or a mezzanine level? Or maybe there was a bar or lounge for the people on this high floor? Sometimes there's a business lounge with free drinks and food for people in executive rooms and suites.

I heard the lift stop and I knew he'd be coming out of it. Apologising profusely, he strode towards me. He looked much older than 50, I'd say late fifties at least, but more than likely he was in his sixties. He was trim, about my height, with short white hair, a smiley face, and he wore a coral polo shirt and jeans.

We then went into his room, which wasn't as grand as I'd expected. It was nice, don't get me wrong, but quite small compared to how I'd imagined it. But the whole side of the rounded room was glass, so the views over the city were fabulous.

He wanted to go straight down for dinner and said we could have a drink in the restaurant, which was fine. As we were about to leave, I contemplated asking for my fee, but decided I'd wait until afterwards. He then remembered himself and pulled out a wad of £50 notes.

I love getting £50 notes. Until I started escorting I had never seen one. They're huge, but because they're not common, when I try to spend them most people are pretty impressed and comment that they've never seen one before. I've never found them difficult to spend, and no one has ever refused one. I do feel a bit embarrassed if I have to try and spend one on a night out, though. If I have nothing but a £50 note in my purse I feel a bit of a dick, like I'm showing off, but sometimes I have to use them if I genuinely don't have anything else. There's nothing more satisfying than looking at a neat £1,000 pile of fifties.

For work they're great, because it means counting the money can be extremely quick. So, the £600 he had given me consisted of just 12 notes, and it took me a matter of seconds to establish it was the correct amount and to tuck it discreetly away. My preference is always fifties.

Trying to count out £1,000 in twenties is a drag, and if it's more, it's a long, embarrassing process. I can't keep talking as I'm counting or I'll lose count, but it feels awkward to be counting and silent. If people pay in twenties, I'd much rather they wrapped and halved one note around four, so they're in bundles of £100 and you can count them without really concentrating.

But I digress. With the money out of the way, we left the room. I was careful not to link arms in case he saw his colleagues. As we walked through the restaurant he was scanning the room for anyone he knew, and I was scanning the layout of the restaurant. It looked expensive, chic and modern. Again, it was all wooden with a full-glass, rounded side.

He decided he didn't want to sit where the waitress initially put us, for fear of seeing his colleagues, so we moved further away from the entrance and tucked ourselves in a window seat behind a small tree.

Our French waiter came over and I asked Colin if he minded me ordering a glass of champagne. He said I could have whatever I wanted, so I asked for a glass of rosé champagne as an aperitif.

Over our drinks we discussed his shooting. He'd shot over 150 pigeons the day before. I joked he'd be having pigeon pie for the next three months! He said he and two of his friends had taken some bottles of wine and cheese, and spent the afternoon getting pissed and shooting pigeons. Now that sounded great fun. I told him about the couple of pigeons I'd shot out of my apartment window, which amused him.

Over dinner he was an interesting and fun companion. It transpired he was separated from his wife and lived in a tiny cottage on the coast with his dog. He had two kids in their twenties, one of whom lived with him.

He said he wanted to know my real name, so I lied and said 'Rachel'. Why do people think that I will tell them my name? If I'd wanted them to know, I'd have used my real name on my website. I used to give it out until two people tracked my address down, one of whom was a regular who ended up threatening me. So now, no matter how long I've known a client, I still protect my identity and often use 'Rachel' as an alternative pseudonym.

I was discreetly checking the time and I knew there was time for dessert, so I wanted to order cheese. Before the waitress had come over to take my order, he mumbled, 'Can't you skip dessert?' We were mid-flow in conversation about something else, so I didn't quite get what he had asked about, but then he added, 'No, that was rude of me, I apologise.' My 'eager beaver' radar popped up.

Then he spotted his work colleagues near the entrance to the restaurant, entertaining some Japanese guys. He kept looking over and I was sure that, contrary to what he said, he actually wanted them to see us because he kept looking and craning his neck, and he passed their table on a trip to the toilet.

Eventually I got my cheese and he'd got himself an espresso and me a mint tea. When I'd finished, he asked if we could go to the room. It turned out he wanted us to leave at the same time as his colleagues so that they did see him – well, 'us'. As he was signing the bill, he made sure he caught the eye of one of them and gave him a wave. I got a kick out of looking at their surprised, but approving faces, and gave them a naughty smile while linking his arm. I knew they'd be gossiping about us.

We had a good hour and half in the room, which was plenty of time. He sorted out the music and I lit my candles and dimmed the lights. In the candlelight, the room looked amazing – out of the window, all the bright coloured lights from the city shone through. He sat in the chair with its back to the glass, and sat me on his knee.

It's quite a buzz to be someone's fantasy; it makes me want to perform and show off like I did in my younger days!

We kissed and I stroked his neck and cupped his face in my hand. To me, touching someone's face is an incredibly intimate gesture, and it's something I do naturally.

It didn't take him long to remove my top, and then almost immediately after, he took off my bra. Why did I bother selecting a nice lingerie set? I could just have worn my day bra, the one with a make-up stain on it, and it wouldn't have mattered. He then turned me back around to fondle my breasts and suck my nipples. Then he lifted me up so he could remove my jeans and knickers. He was directing me, but not in an irritating way – it was quite sensual.

I did get a flashback of the Belle De Jour TV series and imagined I was in it, starring as Billie Piper's character. I had one leg between his and the other up on the side of the chair so he had access to my pussy. He kissed between my thighs and lightly across my pussy and pubic bone, as I looked out over the city lights. It was very erotic.

I pulled his polo shirt up over his head and then he stood to take off his shoes, trousers, socks and boxers. The lot came off in one fell swoop. Bit of a pro, I thought.

On the bed he let me lean back as he licked me softly down below. I wondered how long he'd do it for. Unfortunately it was barely a few minutes before he then straddled me, hinting, with his erect cock in my face. I sucked and licked it, looking upwards at him, he grinned while looking down at me. Then he moved and sat with his back against the headboard and pulled me between his legs so I was sitting upright, but leaning back on him. This was something that lovers would do, and it felt very comfortable and sensual. He had access to both my breasts and down below, and he groped my breasts with one hand and used his other to circulate around my clitoris as I stroked up and down his legs. We sat like this for a few minutes before I lay him on his back and licked up his thighs, gently sucking his balls. He said no one had ever sucked his balls before and he liked it. I love introducing people to new erogenous zones.

I got my bag and took a condom out. He put it on himself and lay me on my back in a rather strange position; so that my head was literally hanging off the bed. It wasn't comfortable at all. I don't know if it was something to do with the fact that he was trying some fancy move that would hit my G-spot or something. After a few minutes I asked if I could put my head up on the bed as too much blood was rushing down and I imagined I must have been beetroot red!

It was clear he had difficulty with the condom as he struggled to keep an erection. At his suggestion, we tried a number of positions. He was trying to force his flaccid penis inside me, which needless to say was impossible. So eventually I took the condom off, wiped him with a wet wipe to get that rubber taste off, and started sucking him again.

It was obvious that it wasn't doing the trick, and my cab was arriving in 15 minutes. So he asked for another condom and fortunately this time he managed to come within a few thrusts. He came and I jumped up, blew my candles out and hastily gathered my belongings from around the room before leaving to catch the cab. I didn't want the taxi driver to be trying to call me and then think I wasn't there and go.

Normally, I enjoy having a kiss and cuddle and wind-down after sex, and because he had taken so long, we didn't have time to do this. So I said my goodbyes, thanked him for a lovely evening and went out to find my taxi.

If I was lucky, I'd be home for midnight. Outside there was no sign of my cab and I was approached by a young black guy asking for my number and if he could come back to Nottingham with me. He asked if I was a student. I didn't know whether to be flattered I looked so young, or offended my clothes made me look like a student! Eventually I got home at 1a.m.

CHAPTER 2:

From Student to Peepshow and Millionaires Island

I have never really been sure what I wanted to do. When I was young, I wanted to be a fashion designer because I've always loved clothes, and I'm very creative.

Many of the designs I did, and ideas I had, came into fashion years later. For example, at 12, I was drawing women in Army-style clothes. This came about because I often went to Army Surplus stores with my brothers, and I wished they had things to fit women, so I drew a series of fitted, military-style clothes. Of course, a few years later this style actually came into fashion.

At 16, I designed platform heels with Perspex, which had been done, but my idea was to put plastic goldfish, hearts or glitter in them, with some glycerine. I got this idea from the snowstorm ornaments that you shake and watch the snow fall. As far as I'm aware, no shoe designer ever created a snowstorm design like that.

At 23, I entered a design competition for Shelly's Shoes. I made a colourful, patterned platform 1960s-style welly from polystyrene and told my family and friends that eventually wellies would be in fashion. They all laughed at me; I was about six years too early for that trend.

In my fifth year at school I was accepted onto an Art and Design Foundation course at Derby University, and at 16 was the youngest there, as most had done their A-levels. On my first day I met Lisa, a girl who was a few years older than me: 21, and very mature for her age. We were very different, but we clicked and spent a lot of time together. But I found it difficult to motivate myself and struggled to stick to deadlines and think of ideas.

Later on that year, I spent most of my time in Belper, smoking pot with my hippy friend Heather and her mates. I had a great time, but I looked totally out of place in hippy clothes, with my make-up and black eye shadow! I passed the year, but hardly with flying colours. After this, I wanted to take a year out, as Lisa was doing, but my parents told me I should get my education out of the way first.

Reluctantly, I went to Wales to start a HND in 3D Design. I got thrown out after the first year for not having done any work, but the course had taken on too many students and I didn't even have my own desk. I couldn't motivate myself, and thinking my lack of study was going unnoticed, I naïvely presumed I could do the same as I did for the foundation, which was to do my work for the whole year a week before it was due in.

For me, living away from home for the first time after a strict upbringing was like a dream come true. Within the first week I had invited the whole college to a kinky pyjama party. About 30 people showed up, and we all ended up licking Angel Delight off each other! My confidence grew because no one bullied me; at college I was accepted.

My exhibitionist side was in full swing and I'd try to shock fellow students. I often went to college wearing a school uniform, tie, over-the-knee socks and a micro mini. Still promiscuous, I slept around with various surfer types.

At college I just wanted to socialise. At the time you're made to think it's a bad thing, but it's only since I've been escorting that I realise it's a real talent to be able to communicate with a variety of people.

I could only get a grant for the degree that I wanted to do if I started that year, so I was unable to take my year out and again reluctantly signed up for a Fashion Design degree in Yorkshire. Really, I should have stayed on for A-levels at school: clearly, I didn't have the motivation to organise myself and get the work done without teachers on my back.

It was in Yorkshire that I met Rob, who became my boyfriend. I went out with him for three months. He was very sweet, but I dumped him after getting bored. The next guy I went out with Richard, I fell for. It was pure lust – I was never in love with him. I had been seeing him for a few months before I found that he had been two-timing me, and he decided to dump me. So I went back to sleeping around. I was bitter because of being dumped and lacked trust in men, so I started being a real bitch to the various older guys I saw. For some reason this made them like me more. That shows how immature I really was at 18 – I have no idea why they put up with me, and I'm ashamed of how I treated them.

Again, all I wanted to do was socialise and at the end of the year, although I passed, I was advised by my tutor to take a year out because I was a distraction to the class and other people weren't working to their full ability because of me. So that was that. It's been a running theme since primary school, when I always had to sit on my own for being a chatterbox. Like most schools the tables were in pairs, and I'd get moved once I started talking to whoever was next to me. I'd think, 'Great, someone new to chat to', so I'd get moved again. They thought putting me next to a boy would shut me up, but it didn't. It was great if it was a boy I fancied. My teachers got so fed up with me that they put two single desks out – one at the front of the class and one at the back.

The really naughty boy in our class got one of them and I got the other!

I moved back home with my parents and flitted from job to job. After having so much freedom, I hated being at home. For a short while I was given the chance to work as a graphic designer for a small local memorabilia business. I had no experience in graphic design, but I put my all into it, came up with some innovative ideas and did everything asked of me without any problems, using all my initiative. It was what I'd been waiting for – someone to give me a chance to shine, and I felt that I was shining.

I didn't want to start at the bottom and work up; I wanted to begin at the top. I was on a basic wage, but I was convinced that if I proved myself, I would earn more. Unfortunately, the main graphic designer left because he knew the company was going under and we were all made redundant. I'd worked for them for just three months. This was a massive knock to my confidence; I didn't feel I had enough experience to go for any other graphic design jobs, so it just became a matter of getting whatever job I could. I did various low-paid jobs – waitressing, bar work and even working in a croissant shop.

When I was 20, shortly after leaving my degree, I bumped into a guy called James in a nightclub. I'd actually met him years before, when he was 12 – he used to come into my dad's shop. I remember thinking at the time that he had real potential, and that in a few years he'd be a real looker. He was 16 when I met him in the club and sure enough, he was absolutely gorgeous. I stopped sleeping around and settled into my first long-term relationship. He was my first love, and as soon as we met, we both fell for each other – I was totally in love and had been swept off my feet. I was terrified. It was the scariest moment of my life; up to that point I had always been in control and had created protective barriers to prevent myself being hurt.

Things were different with James because I had no control over my feelings. He would write songs about me, and poetry, and sing to me; he was so sweet. Our relationship was extremely intense, but also doomed to failure because of our age difference – I was always forking out money for him to get the bus, or buy a bag of chips. He was also very jealous of my male friendships, especially with my ex, Keith, and one of my best friends, Rich. But James used to come to my house on his school dinner break and go back with a big grin on his face. I got some perverse kick out of seeing him in his school uniform! I think his friends were quite envious of him for having an older girlfriend.

He was very insecure, understandably, because of my outrageous dress sense, my age, and also my promiscuous past. In the three years we were together, we had a love-hate relationship. Although I had some of the happiest times of my life, I also experienced some of the saddest. He totally destroyed every bit of my confidence, which I had only just got back after the bullying I endured at school. In fact, probably we both destroyed each other. He was jealous and always assumed I was sleeping around, and we did end up cheating on each other, but I just didn't have the confidence to leave him.

Towards the end of our relationship I started working for an awful, rude Austrian lady as a general assistant at a local hotel, which basically meant I had to do everything, from serving breakfast and cleaning up to cleaning the rooms, checking people out, and opening the bar. It was there that I met a 50-year-old gentleman, Michael, with whom I spent many an hour talking when no one else was in the bar. We became good friends and this was to be my first encounter with someone rich.

He was moving to the US and I accepted an invitation to his farewell party, which was on a barge. For some reason I thought he had invited me there to help by being a hostess, so I dressed in a modest black skirt and white shirt. He turned up in a Jaguar to collect me. My mum was all excited about this E-type Jag, but I didn't have a clue! He was obviously trying to impress me, judging by the smirk on his face as he opened the passenger door. When I got to the car, he was beaming. He asked what I thought, to which I replied, 'It's a bit old,' and 'It's got no seat-belts!' He then informed me smugly that it was an E-type Jaguar, a classic and rare car! 'Oh,' I said, unimpressed.

Obviously I had my wires crossed somewhere and it transpired that I was invited as his guest. I suppose it was like being an escort, really – except I wasn't being paid and he certainly wasn't going to get any sex! It was my first encounter with millionaires. The champagne was flowing, there were caviar canapés and I had a great time, meeting some really interesting people.

Michael then, in his drunken state, suddenly invited me to visit him in the States. I was 22, and had only ever been on a plane once: to visit a pen-friend in Berlin when I was 14. I explained that I couldn't afford it, and he offered to book the flight and cover my expenses. I wasn't sure if he was serious, as I knew he'd had a lot to drink.

The next day, when he sent me a dozen red roses, it was clear he had other ideas about me visiting him. When I told my parents, they were also unsure of his motives, but thought it was a great opportunity. I asked if they could speak with him and his PA, and make it clear that I would go as a friend, no more. He agreed, so we planned to stay at his ex-girlfriend's house in Georgia for three weeks. I spoke with her on the phone, and she seemed pleasant and very bubbly, so I felt reassured.

James, of course, did not want me to go, but I wasn't going to hang about any longer. I knew there was no future with this teenager and I could understand how it made him feel, but the truth was I'd had enough and I was going to do what I wanted to do, because I knew he'd have done the same in my shoes.

I flew out to Georgia, and I ended up having a wonderful time, except that my opinion of Michael changed. I realised he was a control freak and not a nice person at all. What's interesting is that since I've been an escort I've found a lot of rich men are like that because they're used to getting their own way and being able to buy whatever they want, people or products. He was also on a lot of medication, and I suspect he was an alcoholic.

He took me to Millionaires Island, and we spent many nights at 5-star hotels (I had my own room) around Georgia, and dining out at nice restaurants, but I never got to experience the real essence of the place. We only ever stayed in each hotel for one night, and then moved on. We went to Savannah, Jacksonville, and lots of lovely places, but I only ever saw the hotel, and a restaurant. This was my first experience of luxury hotels and I remember thinking I could get used to this life, but it would have been much better to be at these hotels with James or a close friend. It didn't cross my mind that these were the types of hotel I could visit as an escort, because like most people, I thought escorting was seedy and that it was visiting cheap motels for an hour, just to have sex with someone.

One thing I got a real buzz from was driving up to the entrance of these grand hotels, and so did Michael. He loved people to see him being driven around in a sports car by a young blonde and insisted I drove, even though I hadn't passed my test. When we arrived, the valet guy would open the door for me and I'd give him the keys so that he could park the car for us. I always gave my name out and made out it was my car! It made me feel like a movie star. I had never been to a 5-star hotel before, and loved the staff being so friendly and accommodating. Room service was also totally new; I loved the fact that all I had to do was pick up the phone and ask for anything I wanted – food, drinks, fancy cocktails – and a few minutes later a smartly dressed waiter would arrive with my order. All I had to do was squiggle a signature and give him a few dollars. It was mind-blowing! I felt like Julia Roberts in

Pretty Woman, not knowing what to expect or how to behave. Fortunately I didn't have to sleep with Michael, though I'm sure he was trying to impress me, hoping that I would.

The best time I had was when his ex, Anita, took me to Atlanta for a couple of nights and we went out with her transvestite friend to drag shows and a strip club called Guys and Dolls. This was my first experience of such a club and I was in awe of all the dancers. There were men dancing and stripping one side of the club and women stripping on the other. They all took everything off on stage. When a big black hunky man called 'No Fear' stormed onto the stage, wearing Army gear and carrying a fake gun, I squealed with excitement and shoved dollar notes down his shorts at every opportunity! I also loved watching the women and was envious of the attention they got from all the men.

The holiday soured when I crashed Michael's MG. That day, I had specifically told him that I wasn't comfortable driving in Savannah, but he insisted I would be fine. He fell out with me, even though it was his idea for me to drive and he knew I hadn't passed my test, and left me locked in his ex's house as punishment. I called her, crying, and she came straightaway to pick me up. Eventually I was forgiven, but I refused to apologise because I had told him on that occasion that was uncomfortable to drive. He even wanted to go shopping straight after the car had been written off, even though I had concussion and he claimed to have broken ribs.

His comments started to get on my nerves. He said he couldn't stand poor people and made various ludicrous remarks. I constantly put him in his place, because Anita was too polite to, and eventually he tried to send me home. Fortunately, I got on very well with Anita and stayed with her for the rest of my trip. He, meanwhile, moved into his new home.

Meeting Michael made me realise I would never become one of those women who married for money.

While I was away, I kept in touch with James. I knew he

would have assumed the worst: that I was sleeping with this older man. It simply was not true, but nothing I said would convince him otherwise. If I had been happy in our relationship, I wouldn't have gone to America, but the truth was James was making me miserable. When I got back, we still argued and he tried to blame it on the fact I'd gone away, but the problems were there long before my trip; after only six months of being together, we were arguing badly but I hung on, thinking things would go back to how they were, if only I kept working at the relationship.

In the end James left me for someone else, after promising we would get engaged. I only found out through a friend that he'd moved on, but I couldn't accept that it was over and we briefly carried on seeing each other. He promised me that he would leave her and he'd get me to book and pay for hotels so we could spend the night together. I could see there was no spark between us and the times we made love, I left feeling empty and sad because I knew his feelings for me were gone. I was sick of him having his cake and eating it, and informed his girlfriend that he was still seeing me. He said he never wanted to see or speak to me again. So that was that.

Because of my outrageous dress sense, I was getting a bit of a reputation, and in my early 20s I would hear all sorts of stories about myself that weren't true – for example, a taxi driver told my friend's mum that I had been in a porn film. People would make all kinds of negative assumptions about me based on the clothes I wore, but I didn't care. As far as I was concerned, anybody who was a decent person would get to know me and make up their own mind as to what they thought of me.

By the time I started escorting, I'd 'been there, done that' with the whole exhibitionist thing, and now I have a more subtly sexy look. Now I know it's sexier to leave something to the imagination.

My dad has always said to me that I live beyond my means

and he thinks I have expensive taste. Between the ages of 20 and 24, I was earning about £100 a week, and this was simply not enough to fund the things I wanted to do and the clothes I wanted to buy. I remember spending my full week's wages on some red silk and black lace bespoke underwear, which I had made to wear to a New Year's Eve rave at the Pleasuredome in Skegness. As I'd spent so much, that was all I was going to be wearing, apart from some thigh-high patent platform boots! Financially, James took complete advantage of me and was always getting me to pay for hotels so we could spend the night together. Meanwhile, I was still living at home because I could not afford to move out.

Eventually, I found a job with a local travel agent, but I had no experience with computers and was thrown in at the deep end, booking holidays on my first day. Too honest and thorough, I was never destined to get anywhere with the company. I knew I had to move on and I was desperate to make lots of money, but I wasn't sure how.

I knew there had to be more to life and I wanted to do something exciting and different. Being an exhibitionist and loving attention when I was out, I did think that I would love to be a lap dancer.

When one of my friends, Jane, visited from college we took to the stage of the Xanadu night club in Chesterfield for a 'Fake an Orgasm Competition', where we both (and I cringe at this now) decided to try to shock. We did a full-blown lesbian show on a bed – clothed, I might add. All the guys were cheering and egging us on, while the girls looked on in disgust. I loved it. Needless to say, we won and were asked to come back for the final, a couple of nights later.

Arriving, we were approached by a photographer who said he had heard we were the stars of the show. He was eager to catch us in action for a newspaper. Not being as tipsy as the previous night, we simply weren't in the mood, so we passed up the offer of entering the final even though we were set to win. We had thought the prize would be something like an 18–30 holiday, but when we discovered it was a weekend for two in Skegness, we decided it wasn't worth the effort!

I kept in touch with that photographer and he actually took my first glamour photos, which were for a magazine. They were never printed, but I was still paid. Often he would take me and one of my friends to nightclubs around the country, where he was taking photographs.

Another night in Xanadu, I was out with one of my best friends, Tara. We were both dressed in next to nothing – I was in my chain-mail bra, tiny hot pants and chunky boots while Tara wore a tight PVC top with hot pants and boots. Jon, the photographer, was also there and he decided he wanted to take some photos in the club. He took us into the back room, the 'Hollywood Bar', locked it up and we posed together on a grand piano. Lots of faces peered at us through the door and we loved the stir we were causing.

Then we unlocked the door and moved into a back corridor and my friend Rich, the bouncer, and Jon looked on appreciatively as, without prompting, we snogged, groped and ground against each other while Jon snapped away. When we got bored, we went out into the club to dance. The whole floor cleared as though we were an act people had come to see. Everyone stood around the side watching as we groped, kissed and writhed about erotically to the music. We were given three bottles of cheap champagne by the DJ, keen for us to carry on and wondering how far we'd go. Of course, some of the other girls were a bit put out and we did get some drinks thrown at us by the nastier ones. Eventually we left, but we were buzzing from all the attention.

So, after my introduction to the world of glamour photography, I was keen to go to the next step: dancing. I started buying *The Stage* magazine and looking through that with my then best friend, Anna, who was a few years younger than me. She was reliable, honest and I trusted her with my life. Both of us wanted to get rich, have fun, travel and live the high life, with the least amount of effort possible.

I was on flexi-time at the travel agent's and I also worked at a hardware store. I have always been extremely good with people, and whatever job I was doing, even though I wasn't always paid much, I put my all into it. Customer service was, and still is, my top priority: I treat people with the same care and respect that I would like for myself.

Although escorting was mentioned, my friend and I decided we wanted to try exotic dancing, or table dancing, because we thought we would have more opportunities to travel. After spending a lot of time researching, we decided we'd like to go to Japan.

It was then that a spanner hit the works. I'd had arthritis since I was two years old, but hadn't experienced any problems with it since I was 14. Now, though, it was back. I found it difficult to walk, so I started on my medication again, but ended up taking a lot of time off from work because it was too painful to walk. This meant I didn't want to risk going to Japan, so it was back to the drawing board.

After a few months the pain eased and I went back to work, but I knew I would have problems again. However, I was still determined that I wanted to do something different, to explore my wild exhibitionist side and get out of the travel agency, where I had now been for two years, the longest period I had spent working in any job.

I started looking locally to see if there was anything around and found an ad from someone looking for dancers for a club opening in Nottingham. I promptly called, and spent a long time talking on the phone to a pleasant guy called David. I was keen to meet up with him as soon as possible. He mentioned that he was going to the States with his eight-year-old son and I half-jokingly said that I would 'come and baby-sit.'

I became quite good friends with David, although there was

never any attraction there on my part and I did make it clear that I wanted to be no more than friends.

For some time I had wanted breast augmentations and David recommended a guy on Harley Street, someone his ex-partner had used, who had done a good job. I explained that I didn't want to be at home and have it done, so I asked if I could move in with him for a couple of months. He agreed, and so I arranged a loan, left my job, moved in with him and had the operation done. For two weeks I was in constant pain and pretty much housebound. However, it was the best thing I ever did. I had wanted them done for years – I was an A-cup, and so was my mum, so I knew the chances were I wouldn't get any bigger. I'd always loved boobs, and envied ladies with large breasts. I was ecstatic when I saw my new boobs – but they didn't feel like a part of me then, more like two lead weights attached to my front. As time has progressed, they now feel part of me.

David wasn't having much luck in getting a licence for his place in Nottingham, so he suggested that I try working in Antwerp, Belgium, at a peep show his ex had worked at. He took me over for an evening to show me the club. I was instantly offered a job, and given a number to call, if I wanted it.

He then arranged a photo shoot for Anna and me, so that we could have some recent photos to take over to the club. I was really pleased with the glamour-style topless photos. They were taken locally in the woods, much to the amusement of local kids skiving off school.

I got on very well with David's son so shortly after the operation I went away to the States again, this time with David. My friend Anna also went to America with a friend of David's, but the men constantly tried to keep us apart and wouldn't let us speak with each other, so we saw each other for just one day at a water park. We were at different hotels, so we'd call and leave each other messages on the hotel-room phones, but the guys deleted them so neither of us realised the other had tried to get in touch. I had found myself with another control freak, so I ended up disappearing for the last few days of the holiday and booking into a hotel on my own.

Eating on my own one evening, I was approached by a doctor who asked if he could buy me dinner. He was large, in his fifties, with white-grey hair and a friendly, open face. Why not? I thought. We dined and chatted, and I told him that I was going to Belgium to work as a dancer. He then asked me if he could pay for my services. Taken aback, I wondered why he had asked me. In hindsight I realised that a lot of dancers do escorting on the side and you have to be an open-minded, sexual person to do erotic dancing, anyway.

Intrigued, as I had already considered escorting, I decided to press further. I asked what he wanted and he said he'd like to take me to his hotel room, masturbate between my bum cheeks and then clean it up with a wet flannel! A rather unusual request, I thought, as I munched my way through a chicken Caesar salad, but at least he didn't want sex.

It didn't take me long to decide – he was offering me what I was earning for a week's work in the travel agent's. So I agreed, and he paid me $200. I do remember being a little apprehensive that I was going to a hotel with a stranger and no one knew where I was, but I trusted my instinct that he was a nice guy. Besides, curiosity got the better of me.

I was at his hotel for about 15 minutes. Not bad, I thought, for 15 minutes of my time. I didn't even touch or kiss him. The $200 went towards my hotel bill. It seemed so easy! I have always been very open about sex, and to me I couldn't see anything wrong with what I had done.

After that I left the States and never saw David again, thank God!

Shortly after we got back, Anna and I booked our flights to Belgium. I'd told my family I was going abroad to be a dancer – I think I said I'd be doing 'erotic dancing'. They weren't happy about it, because they just wanted me to get a proper job, but there wasn't a lot they could do.

Arriving at the little club in the red-light district of Antwerp, I was extremely nervous, but excited at the same time. I remember it was dimly lit, and there was a bar in the front, with a DJ behind. It looked very seedy. To attract customers, photos of the ladies adorned both the entrance and also a screen by the bar. Various porn magazines and videos were for sale, as well as a large selection of sex toys. A few gentlemen sat perched at the bar, chatting to the barmaid. Then there were all the doors in a circle, with their little windows, and money slots. A man was cleaning the floor with a mop and I realised after my first day at work that he was actually the spunk cleaner. Yuck!

We were taken into the back and introduced to the girls, who came from many different European countries. There was also a couple, who did a sex show on the hour, every hour. We then met the boss, Marc, who was originally from Amsterdam. Slightly chubby, he sported a huge cheeky grin and had short, bleached hair. There was something very sexy about him – when he smiled, his whole face lit up. My friend and I shared an adjoining room with two other ladies. The rooms and facilities were basic, but the accommodation was free so it was to be expected. There were no locks on our rooms, however, and nowhere to keep private or valuable things.

There were about six ladies at work at any one time, along with a couple; also various shifts, starting from 11a.m., with the club closing at 6a.m. for a few hours. Everyone sat in the ladies' room, which was quite large, with comfy chairs, a bathroom and kitchen. Each lady was given a number and took turns to go on stage and perform. The rules were that you had to remove all your clothes and dance; the stage was a large, revolving, round bed with space around the side to walk around. You could touch yourself in an erotic manner, but you couldn't touch the glass windows with the clients behind, and fingering yourself was also considered inappropriate. Each lady danced for three minutes at a time, on average every 15–20 minutes. The shifts were 12 hours long, with one hour for lunch. For this, the pay worked out at about £70 a day.

In between dances, ladies could nip out of the club. It wasn't advisable, though, as they could miss out on getting to do a private show. If a client took a particular shine to a lady, he could request a private dance and this is where you could really make money. No extra cash was made from working the main stage, so it was in the ladies' interests to put on a good show, and hopefully then get to do a private show to top up their income.

Private shows, I was informed, consisted of the lady sitting in a small room with a Perspex screen, which had a small gap in the middle. For most ladies, the private shows on offer were a striptease, pussy show, masturbation show or vibrator show. Prices for these averaged between £15 and £40. My friend was once asked to pee in a cup and put a straw in it, so her customer could drink it! For this, as it was more extreme, the girls advised her to charge £50, which he willingly paid. The prices were for three minutes – if the guy wanted you to stay for longer, he had to put more coins in, or the light would go out and his show would end.

There was a large roll of tissue on the ladies' side, which was slid through the small gap for the gentlemen to clean up any mess.

It was time to begin work, and Anna and I decided to drink a few large vodkas to give us some Dutch courage. I wanted to see what the ladies did on the large, round revolving bed, so when they were called, one by one, I went down the steps to have a look so that I could see what was expected of me.

Generally, it looked quite easy, just sexy dancing and writhing to music. However, I found this quite difficult at first as the music was hard dance! Much to my amusement, my debut was to 'Boom, Boom, Boom, Boom, I Want You in My Room' by the Vengaboys! It's hardly a song to dance to in a sensual manner.

It's strange to hear all the coins in the slots in the booths surrounding the bed and to see the screens coming up, revealing the little faces behind them. There were about 20 booths around the bed in a circle and a guy would go into a booth to watch the show. When he put coins in, the screen would lift up and he'd be able to see the performance through the window. After a couple of minutes, the screen would go down – unless he put more money in, of course.

At first, I felt a bit self-conscious, but I soon became accustomed to it and enjoyed the attention. Some men just looked, others masturbated. I really hated to see them masturbate; at first I thought it was disgusting, but later on, when others didn't, I'd start to wonder why they weren't. Was I not sexy enough? Being involved in the sex trade – day in, day out – made me extremely horny, most of the time. I especially loved the weekends when the club was busy and often full of groups of young lads. It was always a bonus if they were young and good-looking. My confidence grew with the dancing and I was no longer insecure about how I looked.

Often we would get propositioned for sex, but I was earning good money so I didn't feel the need to accept. I could make just as much money simply taking my clothes off and dancing. In a way, I thought doing the peepshow was better than lap dancing because it wasn't so intimate; there was always a barrier between the men and us. Besides, I found it very erotic to have all those voyeurs.

We were in the red-light area, so the guys only had to go next door for a quickie for £40, and it never interested me to take things any further.

After I'd finished at the club, at about 2 or 3a.m., I loved to go to the strip clubs. In my favourite club, the girls would come out onto the bar to hard dance music, strip off their kit and dance round a pole. I was mesmerised and would, and still can, watch them for hours. Then the guys at the bar would lift up the ladies' tops and squirt their breasts with cream. People would pay to lick it off, and I did this many a time!

Once, Anna and I met some English guys there, and because we were dressed in next to nothing (I had on knee-high platforms, tiny denim shorts and a tight pink top), we looked as if we should have been dancing ourselves. The men started paying to lick cream off my boobs, in the same way that they were doing to the ladies who worked there. I got quite a lot of tips! We were also allowed to go on the bar and dance round the pole. Eventually we were thrown out after complaints from the ladies that we were stealing their business, which was understandable, but it was great fun while it lasted.

In the end I guess I wasn't really cut out for peepshow or dance work, because aside from being open-minded, I am also down-to-earth and friendly. In this business there are a lot of jealous ladies, and many have drug and alcohol problems. They saw me as competition – any attractive girl who started working there would be a target for their bitchiness.

It didn't help that the boss took a shine to me, and we started going out discreetly. He was the only guy I slept with during my time in Belgium, as my promiscuity stopped when I was 20 and met James. I was now 23. When he was in the girls' room, I would keep my distance. He wanted me to take days off, and long lunches to spend time with him, but I didn't want to do that, so he'd take other girls out to lunch. Already, I was getting enough bitchiness from the girls. Anna and I drifted apart, and she wouldn't speak to me. She became bitchy, like some of the other girls, while I stayed the same old me.

I was sad to lose her friendship. To this day, I don't really understand what happened. I was upset when she wouldn't speak to me, but she never explained why, even when I questioned her. I wondered if she was jealous of my relationship with Marc, but I always had time for her and wanted to go out with her. We'd had some exciting adventures together and I really missed her friendship.

Sometimes Marc and I would stay away from the club, and he would take me to posh hotels and restaurants. We'd drink champagne, occasionally take cocaine, and visit nightclubs and strip clubs. He was such a funny guy. Every time we checked into a hotel, he would say 'I am Marc,' and as his surname was Schiffer, he would say, '...and this is my wife, Claudia.' With his cheeky face, this always got a laugh and then he would say that he wanted the best room because we had just got married. He would look at me and say, 'Only the best for my darling, eh?' while giving me a beaming smile.

I have one memorable vision of him in a hotel room one evening. Naked, he was jumping up and down on the bed, squashing mosquitoes with a flip-flop. He looked at me with a really serious face, and said, 'See what I do for you, darling? I kill for you!' I couldn't stop laughing – I don't think he realised how funny he was.

I had various problems with my knees, which I knew was inevitable given my history of arthritis. Every couple of weeks, I was paying for a doctor to come out and inject me with steroids so I could go on dancing a bit longer. I had started to get pain in my other joints, and I knew my time as a dancer was coming to an end. Even though the girls could see how bad my knees were, they thought I was skiving off to spend more time with Marc. This was not the case, as I was there to earn money. I was growing tired of some of the bitchiness and competitiveness that went alongside the dance/peep show/ glamour culture.

I spent a total of three months in Belgium before having to return home, much to the disappointment of my parents. I was unable to walk properly as the arthritis had spread rapidly to most of my other joints, and I spent most of the time lying on the couch because my knees were too painful and swollen to walk. Anna stayed out in Belgium, and as far as I know, she carried on with her dancing career and travelled the world.

I was miserable, and quickly became clinically depressed. This was my worst nightmare, as I was not able to have a social life; it was awful. To make matters worse, I had no support from my parents or siblings. They all thought I was exaggerating, and that I was bumming around and didn't want to get a job. Since leaving college, I had never been out of work and the condition I was in, along with not having a job, became unbearable. I felt as though my whole family had deserted me when I needed them most. Even though there were five of us in the house, I have never been so lonely in my life. My sister, who I had been really close to (I had spent many hours advising her about boys and teaching her about sex) decided she wasn't going to speak to me at all for a whole year, and to this day she has never been able to offer me an explanation as to why.

I threatened to report my specialist if he didn't do something quickly. No one likes to be told at 24 'There's nothing else I can do for you', when they can't walk, go out or get a job. I was promptly put on medication I had previously been discouraged from taking, and a date was booked in for me to have an arthroscopy, to see if there was any damage inside my knees. The medication worked, and within a few months I was raring to go. I also needed to decide on my next great plan to make myself rich – I had a bit of catching up to do!

Dancing was no longer an option, so when I saw an ad for escorts in the lads' magazine *Loaded*, I decided to give it a go – I had nothing to lose. It was the perfect time to try because I had no other commitments. I was very blasé and just thought I'd get an ad of my own set up and wait to see who called. As I was going to be working for myself, I knew I didn't have to do anything unless I wanted to. There are not many businesses that you can set up and run yourself, where you don't have to fork out a lot of money initially with no training or qualifications, and where there is such high earning potential. This convinced me that I should give it a go.

It was something I'd already considered when I was looking into the dancing, but as I said, like most people I previously thought it was just like prostitution. When I thought more about it, though, I realised that having been promiscuous I didn't have an issue with having sex with people, and I was single so I didn't have to consider anyone else's feelings. I discussed the idea with friends and they weren't shocked; no one asked me not to do it. Because my friends knew me well, it didn't surprise them – they knew I had the balls to do it, and I think perhaps they were curious, too.

I promptly contacted a company called UK Escorts and was sent an information pack. I decided to go for it and used one of my old glamour photos for my ad, which was online within a few days. It was not an agency as such, because the guys paid the company to view escorts' details, and they then provided them with personal numbers. I had to pay something like £8 a month to be listed, but any money I made would be mine.

By this point my parents were used to my antics. I am so ashamed now of some of the things I said to try and shock them in my teen years – it was very childish behaviour. Of course I didn't think that at the time. In retrospect, I think I just wanted to know how far I could push them, and would they still love me unconditionally?

So when I decided to become an escort, I wasn't about to hide it from my parents. I wasn't nervous about telling them, as I'd told them far worse things in the past. When I told my Mum, she simply shook her head in disappointment and asked me to move out, which was fair enough, and what I had expected. I don't think she was shocked, because for her it seemed a natural progression from the dancing. By this point, I think she despaired of me and my crazy behaviour – I think she really had no hope for me and finally accepted that, much to her sorrow, I was never going to be 'normal', like her three other children.

Diary: July 2008

'Bea wow X' is the name I'm under in Harry's phone. It's quite sweet, really. I've named him 'Harry' as he bears a resemblance to Harry Potter, albeit a bald one, as he shaves his head. He wears glasses and has a young, boyish face. He's single, and in his forties. I suppose he has a geeky look about him, but in a cute way. Often he wears really high-waisted smart cargo pants, with a shirt tucked in. He weight-trains, so in contrast to his cute, boyish face, he has a very manly, muscular, but not OTT body.

The first time I met him was in Rome for a two-night date. Considering he hadn't seen an escort before (so many men lie about this, but he was definitely telling the truth... he really didn't have a clue, and it read all over his face), I thought it very brave of him to book two nights. I have to say it's a bit of a gamble, and I'm not sure that if I was a guy I'd take the risk of going away with an escort for a first date, just in case it turned into a total disaster. On top of that, the cost of the trip and my good self would have set him back a cool £4,000!

I have to confess I'm not the easiest of people to go away with, and for work I'm high maintenance. I can do low maintenance, honest, when it's not for work — as I did when I went travelling to New Zealand and Australia for three months. I didn't even take, or use, a hair dryer or make-up when I was away. However, I was funny about where I slept. Work or no work, I'm fussy about that, but it's because I'm a ridiculously light sleeper. I'm not one of those people who can sleep anywhere, and I hate being woken up or disturbed, especially after a late or heavy night.

But for work everything has to be just so because, mentally, it's the only way I can deal with my job. For work, if I am stopping overnight, I'm very particular about hotels: I prefer them to be a minimum of 4-star. When I stay in a hotel, I like the room to be more comfortable than my bedroom at home otherwise I find it difficult to settle. I like a spacious room, and a massive, comfy bed (I'm too used to my 7-footer at home!), preferably with a large duvet and pillows. There's nothing worse than having a tug o' war during the night with a small, flimsy duvet. I like the room to be comfortable, not too cold or too warm, quiet and with working air con. Yes, I guess I have become rather fussy, but I just don't want the guys I see for work to get a bad impression of me. I'm ratty and horrible if I haven't had enough sleep, so the more comfortable I am, the better night's sleep I'll have, and they'll get the best of me in the morning, too. Knowing this, there have been a number of occasions when I've avoided overnight dates, cutting them short to dinner dates and losing myself £200.

Well, the first time I met Harry in Rome I already knew the hotel was going to be a dive as I'd looked it up on the Internet, and to my dismay it was a humble 3-star. I wouldn't refuse to go just because we weren't going to stay in a 4-star hotel, so I thought I'd make the best of it. Harry reckoned there was a Jacuzzi in the room. It transpired there was a miniscule bathroom off our cramped bedroom, with its uncomfortable, hard bed; and in that bathroom (smaller than you'd get in any budget hotel) was a baby bath, seriously no more than a metre long, with a plastic badge saying 'Jacuzzi'. There were no jets, and the only option was a low pressure shower which hung over it.

Despite the hotel, we had a wonderful couple of nights. He was great company and we saw a few of the tourist attractions, including the Spanish Steps and the Coliseum. We even went to the opera one night. It was fabulous!

Anyhow, back to the arrangements for our date last night... Since his choice of hotel was somewhat shocking in Rome, when Harry suggested a family-run, pub-style 3-star for our trip to Stratford upon Avon, I remembered a friend saying they'd stayed at Ettington Park Hotel and suggested we went there instead. It looked very luxurious, a few miles out of the town in rolling countryside. Fortunately he liked the idea and booked us a suite there for our stay. We also had tickets for The Merchant of Venice.

As my cab from the train station took me out of the small town, through villages to the countryside, I admired the endless green fields and smiled contentedly as we turned up the long, tree-lined drive. I knew as soon as the hotel came into view that it would be as special as I'd imagined. To my right was a large lawn, with a view of a field of sheep in the distance, and I could hear them bleating. In front was a patio, with tables and chairs and a lawn set for croquet. To my left was the gothic manor house that was to be my home for the night.

Turrets towered up high, and the brickwork was various shades of terracotta. There were ornate details on the brickwork and windows. Through the porch I passed a line of wellies, (which is always a sign of a good country hotel), and the staff greeted me with a friendly hello. I hazarded a guess that our room would be up the stairs in front of me, and so I strode up them confidently, seeing an arrow pointing the way to our 'Park Suite'.

Harry opened the door and his eyes lit up. He has a very smiley face, and it was clear he was thrilled that I'd finally arrived.

The room was beautiful and very spacious. We didn't have a king-sized bed, but it didn't matter. There were two large windows with long, thick curtains tied back. By one window was a large round table and chairs; in front of the other was a sofa and coffee table; our bed was on the opposite wall. After greeting Harry, I began admiring our room. It overlooked the croquet lawn and I could see a small chapel in the distance. Right beneath us were the tables and chairs I'd also seen on my way in.

We decided on room service as I'd arrived at 6p.m. and we needed to leave in 45 minutes for the play, so we both ordered Club sandwiches, thinking they should be quick to rustle up. Normally, I wouldn't go for room service on a date but we didn't have long. This was not your average room service, anyway, served in a poky hotel room, eating off your lap and looking out over a car park! We'd be sitting at our own dining table, overlooking the beautiful scenery.

I was disappointed that I'd only been booked for the night, considering I hadn't seen Harry for a year, and I knew he was off work for the whole week. I think he regretted he hadn't booked me for longer, too. He wanted me to stay, but I had a hair appointment arranged for the next afternoon, so I said that for an extra £100, I'd stay until noon.

I know Harry is very comfortable around me. I talk as though we've known each other for years (this is the third time we've met; the second time we went to see England play at Twickenham), and this is one of the reasons I know I make a good escort.

I managed to eat all of my huge Club sandwich, with five minutes to spare. So I went to freshen up in the bathroom and change into the dress I'd brought with me. In the bathroom there was another large window overlooking the lawn. I noticed the bath had a flat-screen TV in it. Nice!

The Merchant of Venice was fabulous. I love getting the opportunity to go to shows and concerts for work; it blows my mind. I didn't know anything about the play, apart from the fact it was written by Shakespeare. I was worried I'd fall asleep, not because I wasn't enjoying it, but because of my short attention span. Normally, if there's no exciting, lively music to keep me alert, I'm likely to drop off. As it happened, I was mesmerised the whole way through.

Afterwards, Harry wanted a drink in the bar. I wasn't really up for it, as I was aware of the time. I was worried that I'd fall asleep. At home, I always go to bed at 10p.m., and that means I can sometimes find it difficult to stay up late when I'm working. Also, I know I need a reasonable amount of sleep, and I know I often sleep badly when I'm working. So, at 10.30 I'd taken one sleeping pill. I got them from my doctor last week, and I had to convince him I would only use them for work, which I will.

My doctor was concerned about me wanting to knock myself out with sleeping tablets because of the nature of my job, which I totally understand, but I am pretty sure that nothing would knock me out that much, and if I ever felt uncomfortable or feared for my safety I wouldn't want to stay overnight with that person anyway.

It was nearly 11.30 by the time we'd returned to the room and I'd lit candles and freshened up. I knew that by 12.30a.m., tablet or no tablet, I'd really need to try to sleep, to get in a reasonable amount of rest.

By the time Harry had freshened up, I was semi-naked, sprawled in a sexy way across the bed in the flickering candlelight. Harry, I knew, would stay up all night if he could, so it was up to me to progress things at a pace that would mean I got to sleep at a reasonable time. He's a rare breed – a lovely kisser – and he complemented me on my kissing. I complimented him back – he probably thought I was just being polite, but he's gentle and not forceful or slobbery in any way.

'Let's take your shirt off,' I murmured. I'd unbuttoned the front, but as he was lying flat, he'd have to lean up a bit for me to take it off totally. 'You've gone all feline,' he murmured back, as he undid his cuffs and removed his checked shirt. 'You're so beautiful, why can't I have a girlfriend like you?' he asked. I didn't know what to say! I asked if he could unhook my bra. He admired my boobs and gently nibbled each one in turn. I reached underneath him and stroked his erect penis through his boxers. He lay beside me and I trailed featherlike kisses down his torso before removing his boxers.

He said he'd taken note when, on our last date, I'd asked why he didn't shave down below if he liked his women shaved. I told him if he liked trimmed, shaved women, he should show the same courtesy, and I smiled and nodded approvingly as I slid off his boxers. He looked pleased as punch.

It's great when men take the time to keep things neat and tidy down below. I'll spend much more time down there if there's no forest of pubic hair. It's so much more pleasant. I love to lick right down in between their legs, down their perineum and up and down their thighs. Also, sucking balls is so much more tempting when they're bald, like little chicken fillets.

Eventually, I lay back and he removed my panties and returned the favour. He has a lovely touch but he has never, during the meetings we've had, spent more than about five minutes down on me. I asked if I should get a condom, and he agreed. First, I lowered on top of him and rode up and down on him, and then we slipped into the missionary position. I clenched my pelvic floor muscles and nudged his hips down with my feet while clenching his buttocks. As he shuddered, I was looking him in the eye.

It was 12.30 when we went to sleep. The sleeping tablets must have worked — I don't remember trying to nod off.

I woke at 5.30 to the sound of heavy footsteps above, and for the next three hours I was in and out of sleep, dreaming heavily. At one point I thought Harry was trying to kiss and cuddle me, and I was pushing him off, telling him to leave me alone. Then it felt as if he was pulling the bed covers down and touching me, violating me in my sleep. I know from experience that this is just a dream, as I often get the same feeling on overnight dates, but when it's happening I don't realise it's a dream. It really freaks me out. I'm scared of going mental and hurting someone by kicking or punching them if I think it's really happening – I need to totally have my own space and can't even bear my leg touching their leg when I sleep, hence my preference for large beds. I guess it's because, deep down, I am worried about someone abusing me in my sleep. But Harry would never do that and I know 100% he wouldn't, so I don't know why I dreamt that he would.

At 8.15 I felt quite awake, so I snuggled up to cuddle him. I couldn't find out if I could change my hair appointment until 9a.m., and breakfast was only served until 9.30, so I thought I should get the morning session going. I gave him oral sex for a short while before suggesting a condom. He wasn't sure it would work, so I suggested he masturbated and I'd do the same. I straddled him and fondled my breasts, and then I pushed my fingers deep into my pussy, and looked at him while licking them. Eventually he gave up, saying it wasn't going to happen. He had been taking some powder supplement for weight training; he said it dehydrated him and he suspected that's why he couldn't come. It bothers me a bit when men don't come…although I try not to take it personally, I feel like I've let them down. But I don't really mind, as long as they seem fine and they've enjoyed the rest of our play time.

I jumped into the shower and when he went in after me, I called to try to change my hair appointment. Fortunately there was a cancellation and I booked for the next day, so we agreed on a leisurely breakfast with a wander round the grounds as the perfect end to our date.

Unfortunately it was raining and although there were wellies, I wasn't too keen to venture out into the cold and damp, so after breakfast we wandered around the house. He asked if the hotel was somewhere I'd like to go for a weekend. Hell, yes! Especially if I could have a spa treatment or two...

A member of staff saw us wandering aimlessly and offered to show us round and tell us a bit about the history. Eagerly, we accepted the guided tour. It was incredibly interesting: it transpired the hotel was over 800 years old, with plenty of controversy, 45 children born out of wedlock, religious conflict and apparently numerous ghosts.

We asked about the chapel and weddings, and I believe the guy thought we were a real couple, actually enquiring about the venue. He suggested an itinerary for our special day, including the ceremony, a blessing in the chapel, the honeymoon suite and their catering facilities. 'He hasn't asked me yet,' I said with a smile, while winking at Harry. They both chuckled, and I think our tour guide wondered if he'd put his foot in it.

After our tour we went back to the room and put the kettle on for a cuppa before we left. Harry spoke about how he wasn't confident with women. He'd tried Internet dating and the first lady he'd emailed had sent him an explicit, legs-akimbo photo after his first contact; it terrified him. The second woman he'd tried to meet eventually confessed that she'd airbrushed her photos and looked nothing like her profile, and she refused to meet him.

One woman he'd asked out at his local gym stopped going. He was convinced it was because of him! I tried to put his mind at rest about that one, saying I was positive that it would have been for some other reason. It made me realise how insecure he was. He, too, was bullied at school, so no doubt that has something to do with it.

I started to explain that I don't like to be directly asked out as it puts you on the spot and you feel you can't say no. I told him one guy had approached me and given me a lovely compliment before walking away, saying, 'I'll be over there, if you want to come and say hello.' I never did, as I was too engrossed in talking to my friend, but I said it's good to express an interest and then leave the ball in the lady's court.

I almost told him to read *The Game*, which is one of my favourite books about an American pick-up artist, who turned from a geek who had zero confidence with women into a full-blown player. Then I thought to myself, 'Hang on a minute, why do I want to do myself out of work?' So, on that note, I left.

Harry walked me down to wait with me for my cab. When it arrived I thanked him for a lovely date, and as the taxi pulled away I matched his sad face, as he waved goodbye. This evening, I'm actually meeting a guy for drinks that I met on a hen do in town on Saturday night. I'm terrified! I can't explain why I'm so confident with men for work and not so in my personal life anymore.

CHAPTER 3:

Meeting the Pimp Daddy

I guess everyone has their perceptions of escorts and escorting, primarily from the way it's portrayed on TV. I think people always assume the worst: there are so many different categories, from £20 prostitutes to the elite £10,000-a-day courtesans. As an escort you set your stall, you make your choices and you set your boundaries. I wasn't about to put myself in the elite category, and I don't remember sitting down and thinking about how much I was going to charge; I knew I wouldn't go for the cheap market. Thanks to my parents and schooling I had good manners, I was well-spoken and I knew I could hold my own and have intelligent conversations with people at all levels. So, I looked at the average prices on the website I was using and set my rates in line with the girls on UK Escorts: £150 for one hour, leading up to £500 for all night.

I had no interest in getting a boyfriend; I'd had my fill of stress and disappointment with James. Now, I needed to be selfish, think about Number One and build my confidence back up. I wanted to have a good lifestyle and have fun without the stress of a man, so I resigned myself to the fact that I'd probably be single for however long I decided to escort. I didn't plan to do it forever – in fact I didn't have any sort of plan, because I wasn't sure what to expect, if I could do it or if I'd enjoy it. I would just test the water and give it a go.

When my first escort ad went online I didn't even see it because we didn't have Internet access at home. I was just sent a printout and told that was how it appeared online. It was strange sitting down and thinking about what services I was going to provide. I remember thinking I wouldn't do everything that I'd done with James, as we experimented a lot, but it was only because we were both so comfortable together. I had many first sexual experiences with James; he always thought I was so experienced and I guess I thought I was too, until I met him. Previously I'd not had a long-term boyfriend – I was never with anyone long enough to get totally comfortable. He opened my eyes to how special and different sex was with someone I cared about.

With James, I experimented with exhibitionism and role-play. One of our favourites is apparently Katie Price and Peter Andre's favourite too – we'd pretend we didn't know each other when we were out. I'd get him to meet me in a pub, in a town where neither of us knew anyone, and I'd already be sitting there, so he'd come over and chat me up. We'd keep it up for hours, even while we had sex, which was usually outdoors; I loved it. I especially loved to play a dizzy, dumb blonde, with a silly, high-pitched giggle. We'd also play doctors and nurses, and indulge in all sorts of role-playing scenarios. I just wouldn't be comfortable doing that sort of thing with a stranger, so I didn't plan to offer anything similar for my escort dates.

So, I had to think about what I would offer as part of my work. I wanted to hold back certain things for my personal life – I knew I could pick what was right for me, what I was comfortable with. I decided that if I didn't kiss, I would feel like a prostitute. It would feel unnatural to be so intimate with someone and not kiss them on the lips. So, I decided kissing would definitely be on the menu. Even though I knew I didn't have to offer oral sex, I guessed I would need to do so to get any repeat business; I suppose that's the thing many guys miss out on at home. I imagined that if I provided this with a condom then it wouldn't be particularly arousing for the gentleman, because I couldn't imagine he would feel much and I'd have to do it for twice as long to make him come! So, I decided to offer this without (OWO), but that CIM (Come In Mouth) would be something I would save for my personal life. Domination, anal sex, humiliation and all the weird stuff would definitely not be on the menu!

I was still at home because I hadn't officially started working yet. And even when I did, I knew Mum would give me a few weeks to sort myself out and find somewhere. She wasn't about to throw me out on the street.

When my ad appeared online, I wasn't prepared for the calls I got. Withheld numbers called me constantly, and dirty old men asked what knickers I was wearing and if I offered anal sex. That was not how I had envisaged things. I was expecting a normal person to call and exchange pleasantries, then ask for my company for a specific date and time. I started to dread hearing the phone ring, so I'd let my answer machine pick up, but no one ever left a message. I was beginning to think the whole thing was going to be a waste of time, but I decided to give it a couple of months before coming up with another plan of action.

UK Escorts warned that I might get approached by television companies. When I did receive a call, I was naïvely excited! I felt honoured to have been called, and once they found out that I hadn't yet done an escorting job, they thought showing the beginning of my career would be perfect for their programme. Their idea was to show the glamorous side of escorting, to try to dispel the 'escort = prostitute' myth. They wanted to feature a series of ladies going about their work, preparing for dates and organising their business – to show that they were sound-minded women with a good head on their shoulders. So, they did a series of interviews about what I thought about escorting and why I had chosen to do it, and they were keen to capture my first job.

Being followed around felt very important and I loved the attention and gossip caused in my small local town by me having a TV crew following my every move. Soon, the local paper had a front-page story, which they had to improvise because no one knew what was going on. This must have been an embarrassment for my dad at the newsagent's, as the local paper was displayed with the heading REBECCA'S NAKED AMBITION stamped on the front page. It claimed I was going to be an international glamour model (I wish!), and someone had kindly provided all the details of where I went to school and college.

I still had no escort work: I could have taken some on, but I wanted to wait for proper gentlemen to call.

It transpired that on one day of the filming, my debut appearance in a UK magazine was out for sale on the top shelves. Ironically it was the magazine *Escort*, which has nothing to do with escorts. It was one of a few glamour jobs I managed to do before I went abroad. The film crew loved this and followed me round on a mission to get a copy.

But I couldn't find a copy anywhere. Naïvely, I thought that no one locally would find out about it. I went to my next local town and the newsagent told me they had sold out. He said that the magazines had flown off the shelves and that he had more on order, and he asked if I was the lady in the photos. I ended up having to go out of town to find a copy. When I saw it, I cringed. It was a two-girl shoot, the theme being 'moving in', and both of us ended up in various shots with plastic buckets of clothes!

Three months after my ad appeared online I received my first voicemail. It was from a guy called Ade, who said that he ran a listings site where girls were earning £2,000 a week. I thought he was exaggerating, but was interested to meet him because I still hadn't arranged any work. We met locally and he showed me colour photocopies of the ladies on the site. There were about ten in all at that time, and now there are over 100! He also let me speak to a couple of women on the phone, and I was quickly convinced that I had nothing to lose by giving it a go.

Then came the snag: I was told that every now and then he liked to meet up with one of the ladies, take her out for the evening and spend the night with her. It was obvious what he wanted. I remember thinking, 'So, this is what a pimp looks like'. He wasn't at all what I was expecting: he was in his forties – small, balding and average looking. He looked like a timid little salesman. There was no big fur coat or 'bling'!

I got a bit short with him, argued my case, said what he was proposing was unreasonable, and left. He had offered to give me three months' free listing to prove the site would work for me. Normally, it would be £40 a month. However, if I didn't sleep with him, I would have to pay £300 a month. Later, I found out that I was just his type – blonde and slim, with big boobs. He didn't ask everyone, only those he fancied and those new to escorting, or who were young and didn't know any better.

I don't like things being expected of me and I felt cheated. He emailed me to tell me, in a roundabout way, that because I wouldn't sleep with him, I was unsuitable.

I thought about the situation a lot. At the end of the day it was my choice and I know now that had it not been for him, I might not have had the successful business I have today. I decided the good points outweighed the bad: I needed money, so to me it would be like a practise run for the real thing. I'd find out if I could really do it, and if it turned out I couldn't,

I wouldn't actually lose anything. I emailed him back and told him I'd changed my mind.

He was dubious at first, but then he arranged to meet me for an evening in Manchester, which involved him taking photos of me to put on the website, followed by dinner out and then a bit of sex at the hotel in the evening, and again in the morning. Really, it was a practise run for an overnight booking, as he was an average looking businessman in his forties.

Doing the photos was fun, and I had lots of ideas for what I wanted to do. The shoot was a success, as was the evening that followed. We had dinner and then we went to a lap-dancing club, where he paid for me to have a couple of dances with the ladies. After that, we went back to the room and had foreplay and sex for a couple of hours. Then I knew I was up for the challenge of being an escort. It all seemed so easy! Sleeping with strangers was nothing new to me because of my promiscuous younger days, so it really wasn't a big deal to have sex with him.

I didn't have to consciously detach myself from the experience. I just knew this was someone that I didn't know or care about so there was no feeling in my head or heart when I had sex with him; I simply had fun and made the best of it. I have always got a buzz out of giving people pleasure. Even before my escorting days, I always put the man's pleasure before my own. That's probably why I've never had an orgasm through penetrative sex.

Ade advised me on what to charge, and after hearing his stories about the girls on the site, and realising that escorting could be like going on real dates if I wanted it to be, I knew it was for me. To get paid to eat and socialise, what could be better? This was when I first heard the term 'Girlfriend Experience' (or 'GFE') which is, as the name suggests, being paid to be a 'girlfriend' and companion for the evening. I was keen to specialise in the longer bookings that included dinner, because it would be like going on a real date.

Ade advised me to charge £250 for one hour, which at the time was a lot for the north of England, but it's to discourage people from booking just an hour. Every hour after that was an extra £100, and an overnight date would be £700. I couldn't think of a name for myself, so when he suggested 'Barbie' (because I was very girly and liked pink things at the time), I couldn't think of anything better so I went along with it.

My dad's advice was to contact the Inland Revenue and register as a self-employed escort, to organise paying National Insurance and also to get myself an accountant. He recommended the family accountant, who hadn't a clue about escort accounts, but he took me on. That all sounds ridiculously practical, but I think it was just my dad's way of dealing with it. He didn't want to talk to me about my escorting – it's not as if he didn't care, but he just didn't know what to do with me. My parents never thought it would work out, and I think they hoped it would just be a short phase and thought that if they left me to it, I'd be back eventually with my tail between my legs.

CHAPTER 4:

My First Date

Date: 04/08/2000
Day of the Week: Thursday
Time of Day: 7p.m.
Time Spent: Overnight
Price: £700
Place: Met at my home in Liverpool
Description: Barbie is a natural blonde, with – wow – natural breasts and a firm, amazing body. She is slim – size 10 at the most.
Comments: When Barbie arrived, we went straight out for dinner at a local French restaurant. Her pseudonym 'Barbie' does not do her justice, as despite her babe looks, she is certainly no bimbo. I found that her fun, sincere and intelligent personality made for a very pleasurable evening. After a relaxing dinner, we returned to my apartment, where we played a sexy version of 'Spin the Bottle', ending up with both of us stripped naked. This was girlfriend sex at its best. My date with her was one of

the most erotic and sensual experiences of my life. I've seen quite a few escorts in my time and I've seen some of the best around, but Barbie is up there with them. She's number one in my book! To be the perfect escort, it takes a very special woman and I have found that in Barbie.

I believe that because of the combination of her looks, personality and sexuality she will be a very sought-after lady. Guys, get to see her while you can because they don't come any better!

Even before I had my photos on the website I received a call for an overnight booking in Liverpool. Ade had contacted a guy who regularly saw the ladies on his site and had given me a glowing report, following which the guy insisted he saw me the very next day.

I broke the news to Mum and Dad that I was embarking on my first escort job and that it would be in Liverpool. They knew about the listings site, but obviously they didn't know that Ade had asked to sleep with me. To put their minds at rest, I truthfully told them that this particular client had seen loads of girls and was really nice, and that he'd booked us a table at a French restaurant. Neither of them tried to talk me out of it, they just accepted it – which is all they could have done, really. I think they were hoping that I'd learn from my own mistakes, and maybe that I wouldn't enjoy it and could then move on and get a proper job. Mum agreed to give me a lift to the bus station, and I said I'd leave them full details of where I was going and who I would be visiting. They didn't ask me to do this, but I knew they would worry, so I decided I'd give them this information for every job I went on, for my own safety as well as for their peace of mind.

I called my friend Nat and gave her the exciting news. She wanted me to phone her as soon as I got back and give her all the juicy gossip!

So this was to be my first escort job. I was thrilled and excited, not nervous at all. I think this was mainly due to the fact that I'd had lots of reassurance from Ade about the guy – he'd seen so many girls and obviously Ade had had positive feedback. He was the perfect candidate to break me into my chosen profession. Had the booking come in from someone that Ade didn't know, I think I would have been terrified.

It took me about two hours to prepare for the job. I think I was also subconsciously readying myself mentally; I wanted to look preened to perfection for him so I spent a long time bathing, shaving, moisturising and doing my nails.

I picked out black, sheer lingerie with delicate pink bows. For a long time, I deliberated about what to wear, going through the garments on my rail, all of which were clubbing clothes. I wasn't about to wear my hot pants or rubber dress, and I didn't have any skirts or dresses that were on the knee or below, which left trousers as my only option. Most of mine were funky, tight, boot-cut flares. I had a leather-look pair and a snake-print PVC pair that I wore all the time. In the end, I decided on the leather-look, which I wore with some black platform boots, a tight black top and a dark denim jacket. I just didn't have any ladylike clothes – I didn't do ladylike. I did chunky and funky club wear.

Before arriving for the job, I decided that I wasn't going to think or worry about it. I was surprisingly confident. As someone who genuinely enjoys meeting all sorts of people, this was the part I was looking forward to. I knew that I was being paid for my time and that most of that time would be spent socialising, something that came naturally to me, and I think that was mainly why I wasn't nervous about my date. And of course, having been promiscuous, I wasn't worried about the sexual side of things.

One thing that I couldn't help but think about was how to make the move to the bedroom after our meal. I still wasn't sure, but decided to go with the flow. Being the chatty, open person I am, the conversational side of things didn't bother me at all. I knew I would be OK.

I had a 40-minute bus journey and then caught the train to Liverpool. The journey took about four hours. When I arrived at his house, I took a deep breath, put on a big smile and rang the doorbell. He invited me in – he was an accountant, average looking and in his forties, with glasses, dark hair and a medium, trim build. He looked like your typical accountant. I remember thinking, if they all look like this and they're all as easy-going as this, the job will be easy!

We went straight out to a nearby French restaurant. The meal was very tasty and the wine flowed. I couldn't believe that I was being paid to go out for dinner with someone at a posh restaurant! I was totally overwhelmed by the whole experience. It was so exciting, I loved it! Thankfully he didn't seem to mind my clumsy choice of attire.

Back at his house, we had a further drink and I suggested a game of strip spin the bottle, which made for a smooth transition to the bedroom.

I actually found it a quite a buzz that this guy was so in awe of me and willing to pay so much money just to be with me. We spent about an hour or so undressing and caressing, and giving each other oral sex. I was a bit of a show-off. The more he looked at me appreciatively, the more it made me want to perform. I wanted to be his ultimate fantasy. So, I writhed on the bed and teased him, looking up at him in a coy but suggestive way. I then straddled him and let his hands wander over my body. I used the tip of his penis to rub my clitoris, while I squeezed my boobs together to maximise my cleavage. I've always understood that men love visuals and women who are confident with their bodies.

I wasn't sure how long we should indulge in foreplay and I didn't know how long this guy was going to take to come when we had sex, or whether I should offer the condom or wait for him to ask. Eventually he asked me for one. My bag was in the other room! There's a learning curve, I noted to myself. So, I had to pause our playtime while I jumped off the bed, rushed out of the room to find my bag and fished about for a condom... all the while praying he'd still keep his erection! Once I had found one, I went back to the bed and sucked him again to get him back to his full erection before slipping on a condom, and getting on top of him. By this point he was so excited that he didn't last very long at all.

About 1a.m., we went to sleep and in the morning we had a bit more sex, this time with less foreplay, before having breakfast. He said he really liked me and that he would want to see me again, and then he paid me cash in twenties: £700. I couldn't believe it! I had never held so much money in my hand before and I couldn't stop grinning. I was beginning to feel as though this job was my ticket to getting rich and living the lifestyle I had dreamed about. A couple of months later he helped me to sort out my mortgage by confirming that I would have no problem making the payments, and we estimated how much money I would make for the year.

On the train home, I sat with a huge grin on my face, discreetly clutching the envelope in my bag and staring out the window, thinking, this is it – I'm finally on my way up! I daydreamed about what my life would be like: I'd be one of those glamorous women in designer clothes, with perfect nails and hair, designer handbags and shoes, breezing in and out of posh hotels and restaurants, with slick businessmen taking me all over the world... First-class travel... Paris...

I rang Nat and left her a long, rambling voicemail about how I had found it so easy, and that I was buzzing and had £700 in my bag!

The first thing I did when I got home was to count the money, and put all the Queen's heads the same way, so they were neat. Then I counted it again... and again, before tucking it away back in its envelope. When Nat eventually called after she'd finished her boring 9–5 job, the questions rolled in:

'You got *how* much?'
'What did he look like?'
'How old was he?'
'Were you nervous?'
'Where did you go to eat?'
'What was the sex like?'
'Was it difficult?'
'Did you fancy him?'
'Are you going to see him again?'

She was proud of me and said she could never do escorting. I remember thinking, it's no big deal, really... but I guess to most people it is.

Date: 18/19 November
Day of the Week: Sunday/Monday
Time of Day: 8p.m.
Time Spent: 2 overnight stays
Price: £1,400
Place: My hotel
Recommended: Yes
Would You Return: Yes
Description: The photos on Barbie's page are excellent, but don't do this beauty justice. She's around 5'8" with heels, and platinum blonde hair. Her figure is fabulous... she's a real STUNNER!!!!

Comments: I contacted Barbie easily by phone, and had a couple of phone conversations. She likes to weed out timewasters and after a couple of calls, a date was arranged. When Barbie turned up at my hotel (bang on time) I couldn't believe my eyes. What a babe, she is absolutely gorgeous!
   Barbie confided in me that she was training to be a masseuse, and I was invited to her college as part of our

date as she needed a volunteer to practice on. A relaxing massage was the perfect start to our overnight date! I was after the famous GFE, 'Girlfriend Experience', and Barbie offers this to perfection: lots of attention, lots and lots of love and tenderness, and forever asking if I was OK. Yes! What hot-blooded male wouldn't be?

Barbie has it all: the personality, looks, brains and sense of humour. She is an absolute joy to be with!

Guys, I am not going to go into the sexual side of things – all I will say is that I went home a very satisfied, content and happy man, the pinnacle of our time being bringing her to an orgasm on our second evening. There was no fake moaning and groaning here, this was for real!

You have to be prepared for people staring at you as a couple because of her drop-dead gorgeous looks. I enjoyed this immensely!

Barbie prefers the longer dates, rather than the two-hour 'wham, bam, thank you, Ma'am' because she likes to get to know people. This isn't her being greedy – she is just a very special lady who is very good at her job.

I can only say I wouldn't spend £1,400 on just anybody! I will be seeing Barbie again in January, and this will be my one and only review, gentlemen, as I can assure you, if you meet her you won't want to see anyone else either! Thanks, Barbie! Roll on the New Year!

CHAPTER 5:

Embracing the Role

After my first job, the ball was rolling. I was buzzing and confident because of how well it went and how easy it was for me. So, when the overnight enquiries came in, I loved it. I started getting reviews on Punternet (a review site for escorts and working girls). They were all for overnights, so overnights became my thing. People would read the reviews and only book me for overnights. This was perfect, but it wasn't a case of only wanting overnights because they earned me more money. They also take up a hell of a lot of time. For overnight dates, I travel all over the country and to Europe. Even for jobs in this country, I can be out of the house for over 24 hours.

I could actually make more money and use less time if I did short bookings and in-calls, but to my mind this would just be prostitution. It was years before I did my first one-hour job and I haven't done many at all. Four one-hour calls could make me the same amount of money as an overnight, but I enjoy the travel, the different hotels, restaurants and scenery.

Being a people person and genuinely enjoying meeting new people, I knew I wanted to get to know the guys I met, not just spend time in bed with them. I have friends in the business who prefer the opposite. They don't want to socialise with their clients – they just want to have sex with them and go.

My overnight work kit is all packaged up in an innocent-looking vanity case. The bottom layer has all my wash stuff and normal toiletries, and then on the top part, I have my 'work kit'. Over the years, this has changed and been adapted as new products come onto the market and I learn from my mistakes. Presently, my essentials for work are: condoms, lubricant, a vibrator, massage oil and candles. Then there are overnight essentials: my eye mask, snore strips (they really work because they open the nasal passage at the top of the nose!), my ear plugs (essential for noisy hotels and snoring), and nowadays I take a plug-in to fill the room with eucalyptus, as further reinforcement against snorers.

I know all this sounds ridiculous. Think how sexy I look with my earplugs in and eye mask on! Some of the guys I see think it's hilarious when I get ready to sleep. At least it saves me being disturbed if they get any sexual urges in the night: one look at me in that get-up kills the moment more quickly than an image of their granny naked!

One night I had a few sniffles when I was with a client and we both had nasal strips on. In the morning, we just looked at each other and laughed. We looked like a pair of Moomins!

These days, I still get as much of a buzz out of being in a posh hotel or restaurant as I did when I first started escorting. I have to admit, although I'm really a country girl at heart and love weekends on my uncle's or granny's farm, slobbing around in jeans with no make-up, drinking beer and listening to my brothers play acoustic guitar, I love the opulence of my work as it's such a contrast. Around 99% of the time I visit 4- and 5-star hotels, but I've also been to some beautiful homes. I still can't comprehend people spending between £500 and a £1,500 a night on hotels. Personally, I couldn't justify that kind of money – well, maybe I could if I was mega-rich!

I once met a guy in London who'd booked the penthouse suite. It had two bedrooms, three bathrooms, a huge lounge and a dining area. Seriously, who needs *three* bathrooms? It was four times bigger than my spacious apartment in Nottingham. But I'm certainly not complaining; times like that, I think 'This is the life!'

My favourite overnight dates are those when I get to watch some sort of concert or show, when I'm spending time with one of my favourite chilled regulars. To me, this is what offering the 'girlfriend experience' is all about.

Diary: August 2008

Thornbury Castle was my idea. I was to meet Peter for a country-house break, away from his busy work. He suggested somewhere in south Wales, but that would have taken me five hours on the train. Having said he was open to other suggestions, I asked around on the escorting forums online and Thornbury Castle was mentioned, so I sent him the link, along with a few others.

He wanted to stay at Thornbury as he said that Henry VIII had stayed there with Anne Boleyn. We'd never met before and, as I have said before, I always think it's a brave thing for a guy to do – book two nights away with someone he's never met.

The hotel looked absolutely amazing. He'd booked us in to see Henry V, an outdoor performance in the Tudor gardens on the Friday. We had an hour and a half of clay pigeon shooting booked for Saturday afternoon, and I had a facial arranged for teatime on the Saturday.

The date had been arranged about six weeks in advance, which is just how I like it. I prefer my diary to be organised in advance so I know what I'm doing and when; it's easier for me to plan my finances.

Closer to the day we liaised about what clothing to bring and I said I'd arrive in smart jeans, if that was OK with him, and I'd wear them that evening for the outdoor performance. I'd take a dress for the next evening, and I'd bring my wellies and waterproof as the weather forecast had given out showers. He got back to me and said it was all fine.

Twenty minutes before the cab was due on the Friday, before I'd even dried my hair and was rushing about, panicking like a mad woman, he texted me to say that he'd arrived and that the hotel was very formal.

I didn't know what to do, and I started worrying. Did he now want me to bring different clothes? He wouldn't text me if he thought that what I'd planned to bring was OK, would he? I decided I'd wear my white jeans for travelling instead of my dark blue ones (thinking they looked a bit smarter), and threw in a summer skirt and top for the evening performance. Barefaced, I rushed out with my suitcase and threw my make-up in my handbag to do on the train.

Thankfully, all my trains were on time and I jumped in a cab at Bristol Temple Meads without having to wait. When the driver found out where I was going, he commented how fabulous and expensive it was. 'Someone's treating me,' was all I offered.

We drove out of the city and into the countryside. Eventually we reached the little town of Thornbury, which was more like a small village. As we pulled into the long drive, there were fields either side of us and the big stone walls of the castle. Someone was just leaving in a helicopter and we had to wait a few minutes for it to take off. As we drove through the entrance into a courtyard, the castle looked fabulous.

I was dropped off at Reception to be greeted by a young guy. I told him my partner, Mr Hartswood, had checked in. He said, 'You must be Miss Barratt?' and it took me a few seconds to realise that I had used that name when I booked the spa treatment. I always use the name Barratt if I need to book anything. 'Shall I call him, or would you like to surprise him?' he asked. Er... surprise him,' I answered dubiously. He took me across the courtyard and I saw someone walking towards us. I guessed it was Peter, and as the gap between us closed, I could see he was smiling. I smiled back, hoping I looked like this was my partner and not someone I'd just met for the first time. Peter was quite small and chunky; he looked around 35, with lightly freckled skin and fair, cropped hair.

The guy came with us and took my heavy case up the winding stone steps to our room, where there was a massive oak door with a metal latch. It creaked open and the porter took in my case and left us to it.

I was so excited. The walls were stone and we had a curtained four-poster bed. It looked just as I imagined it would have done all those years ago when kings and queens visited, apart from the TV and modern bathroom. On the side was a decanter of sherry and various pieces of old dark wood furniture and deep, red chairs. The ceiling was very ornate and carved, and there was a fireplace on one side of the room; the bathroom was cosy, with marble fittings and gold taps.

Peter said he'd taken the liberty of booking us in for the pre-show dinner at 6p.m., but I'd arrived at 5.30, so there wasn't much time to get ready. On top of the TV were some bottles of water and a glass jar of homemade biscuits. I asked if I could have one, which he said was OK. I took a bite of it, and walked towards him. I'd barely entered the room and we'd never met before, but he pulled me close and closed his eyes, even though my mouth was obviously full of biscuit and he'd seen me bite into it. I thought, 'He can't seriously want to kiss me right at this moment, surely?' But he did, and not only that, he went for the full-on snog, leaning in with his eyes closed and mouth opening. Now I'm all for sharing, but...! 'I have a mouthful of biscuit!' I exclaimed, jerking back from him and covering my mouth to avoid spraying him with crumbs. 'I'm sorry, I sometimes do stupid things,' he muttered. Oh dear, what had I let myself in for?

I put on a little more make-up and asked if I could go to the outdoor performance in what I was wearing. He said yes. I was wearing boot-cut, smart white jeans, a gold belt, nude heels and a sloppy, smart fawn Chloé T-shirt with gold jewellery. I put my raincoat and sweater in my bag – I was pretty sure it would rain.

The castle was a warren of rooms with various dining rooms and lounges. All were adorned with traditional furniture, some had dark wooden walls and tables, and there were old paintings of kings and queens, plus various tapestries. The food had all been produced locally and was delicious. Over dinner it transpired my date didn't like vegetables or fruit, and he confessed that he only had takeaways at home, which explained his somewhat pasty skin and chunky body. He let me choose the wine and I picked a bottle of Sancerre to accompany our meal. There was a Manuel-style old waiter, who constantly went around fussing and topping up all the tables' wine and water, even when it didn't need doing. His suit was crumpled and dirty, but he was very sweet.

Just as we were finishing our teas, a dark cloud came over and the room plunged into darkness. I knew we were about to get soaked outside. It had been sunny all day, it was Sod's law!

As we left for the performance it started to rain. We picked up a large umbrella from the hotel foyer and made our way to the Tudor garden. Plastic seats were set out and most people were already seated. A few huddled on the ground and tried to keep the rain off with umbrellas. This would be quite an experience!

The performance started, and again I was mesmerised by a Shakespeare play. Even as the rain got progressively worse, the actors never faltered. At times we couldn't hear a word they were saying as the rain was torrential and Peter, bless him, held the umbrella throughout the whole performance. The actors were getting soaked, but seemed oblivious. They gave it their all and in true British style everyone stayed put for the duration. There was an interval and we managed to get a cup of hot chocolate to warm us up before the second half.

After the performance, we made our way to the bar, even though we were drenched. I ordered a vodka and he had a pint of lager. He had obviously chilled out since the earlier attempt at the biscuit snog – I had expected him to want to go to the room, but as it happened we had three drinks in the bar before retiring at around 11.30.

We put the fire on when we got back. Although it looked like a real fire, thankfully it was gas, so we had a bit of heat straightaway. I jumped into the shower to warm up and came out snug in a luxurious robe. He got up and moved towards me, grinning as he leant down to kiss me, slipping his hand inside my robe to grope my breast. We moved to the bed and he wasted no time in getting naked. I slipped off my robe and he pushed me gently back on the bed, kissing me and moving his mouth down my neck to my breasts and then briefly to my pussy. He was one of those guys who avoided my pubic area, apart for a couple of gentle kisses.

He then lay beside me and I straddled him, kissing his mouth, neck and down his torso. I took his erect cock in my mouth and sucked him for a few minutes until he asked if I had a condom. I reached for my bag and slipped one on him. We spent a few minutes each on top, and he silently climaxed quickly while he was on top. 'Did you come?' he asked. 'Er, no,' I answered.

He rolled off and went to the bathroom. When he confessed he was a snorer, I put a snore strip on his nose. I'd had two of my sleeping tablets, so I was ready for a good night's sleep, but no sooner had the lights gone out than he started snoring, very loudly. The strip wasn't working at all! Eventually he said he'd move to the small two-seater sofa. I was half-asleep. He continued to snore, but the bit of distance between us helped, although I still had a restless night.

I woke about 8a.m. and looked across the room. Naked on the sofa, he looked most uncomfortable, but as he'd snored all night I knew he hadn't had a problem sleeping. I was extremely envious that he could sleep so easily! Breakfast was served until ten, so I suggested we order room service, but he wanted to go down to the breakfast room. Shattered, I didn't know how I was going to get through the day.

We ordered coffee and tea, and a cooked breakfast. Our clay pigeon shooting lesson was at 1p.m., so we had time to shower after breakfast.

I assumed he'd want some morning fun, so I showered and left my robe on, but he got dressed so I did the same. I left my mud-splattered jeans at Reception for them to wash and return from the laundry later in the day — I didn't have anything else apart from the denim skirt I had on.

At the shooting range we were kitted out with shooting jackets, glasses and baseball caps, and had a short introduction on how to hold the gun. He'd never shot before, but I had on the family farms, so I knew how to stand, hold the gun and shoot.

The instructor kept referring to me as 'Mrs Hartswood'. I find it odd that in this day and age people automatically refer to you as husband and wife, which they especially seem to do at hotels. He was very impressed with my shooting skills and Peter, once he got the hang of it, was an excellent shot, too. We shot a variety of clays, including the 'rabbit', which came out and rolled across the grass! I was particularly good at that one. Our instructor pressed on, giving us more and more challenging shots. We both shot about 60–70% of the clays each, which considering it was Peter's first time shooting clays and my second, was rather impressive.

Both of us thoroughly enjoyed the afternoon. Peter asked what I wanted to do, and if I wanted to go to a pub after, but I fancied having a champagne afternoon tea in the garden at the hotel, so he said we'd do that, even though he thought it was a bit 'wot, wot' – he meant posh.

It was a beautiful day, so we sat in the castle grounds with champagne, tea, and an array of finger sandwiches and cakes. Perfect. The waitress asked if we'd like to book a table for dinner, but much to my disappointment he wanted to go out for a Chinese or

Italian meal. I guessed this was because he could avoid the vegetables! So, the hotel booked us into a local Italian for 8p.m.

At about 4p.m., he asked if the sun made me horny. I replied that it did, so we finished up and made our way back to the room. He wanted me to keep my pink wellies on! So we had a quickie and I rode him with my skirt and wellies on. I think he got a kick out of it – the 'farmer's naughty daughter' scenario, perhaps.

I had a facial booked in the room for 5p.m., and he agreed to let me have a couple of hours on my own, so he left with his paper. He left me £60 to pay for the facial, which was kind of him. Sometimes guys can be too clingy when you're away for a couple of days, but thankfully he was very chilled and I was enjoying my time with him.

The facial was wonderfully relaxing, but I didn't sleep as I'd hoped and by the time I'd got myself ready for a snooze, Peter came back. We both showered and got ready for the evening. It was too cold for my skirt and the dress I'd brought would have been totally over the top for the local Italian, but luckily my jeans were back from the laundry.

We couldn't get a cab, but someone from the hotel offered to take us, and when a black Bentley arrived at reception, I felt a twinge of excitement. This is what my job's all about: the glamour, I love it!

We pulled up outside the restaurant and I could see people craning their necks at the window, obviously wondering if Posh and Becks would be stepping out! I felt like a VIP.

Pondering what to order, I told Peter I'd had far too much bread that day. 'As long as you don't say "D'oh"!', was his reply. Oh dear! He started babbling and making rubbish jokes, which he thought were going over my head, but they just weren't even mildly amusing. Lack of sleep was clearly starting to get to me. I could feel myself becoming really wound up and irritated because I was so tired and my eyes were welling up. 'Please don't cry,' I silently begged myself.

I escaped to the loo for a few minutes to try and pull myself together. There, I switched on my phone as I had to text my auntie to let her know what time to collect me the following day (my aunt, uncle and cousin live near the hotel, so I was going on to see them). I took a few minutes to compose myself by closing my eyes and taking a few deep breaths.

Back at the table I decided I didn't want a dessert, but he ordered his favourite, Tiramisu. He kept asking me if I wanted some and I got a bit snappy because he did this three times. Peter was drinking beer and I'm sure this makes some guys snore all the more, so we discussed what we were going to do that evening to combat the problem. He said his nose had been broken a few times and that's probably why he snored. 'I could stuff your nostrils with cotton wool,' I suggested. He looked at me strangely, probably wondering if I was joking. But I really needed a good night's sleep and I started worrying that I wasn't going to get one. He kindly said he'd sleep on the sofa again. Now that's a genuine girlfriend experience, or maybe a WFE (wife experience)! I suggested he gave me a 20-minute head start to allow me try to get to sleep, so that's what we arranged to do.

Back at the hotel he kindly said that I could go to the room and sleep, if I wanted, but I offered to go to the bar with him. I found a box of cards and taught him how to play 'Shithead'. The card playing, combined with the double vodka, perked me up a bit. Together, we left for the room.

Back there, he wanted another quickie (quickies seemed to be his thing and I wasn't about to complain!), so I put on a sheer set of lingerie with the hold-up stockings he'd requested, and we had a session before bed.

He left to get comfy on the sofa and I covered him in a blanket. Then I got some cotton wool from the bathroom and stuffed both of his nostrils with as much as possible. I couldn't help but laugh! Fortunately it worked and I had a much better night's sleep. I was still in a deep sleep when he shook me to wake me. I woke with a fright and almost jumped out of bed – it was 9a.m.! Normally, I don't lie in, but I think I was catching up on my lack of sleep from the night before. I was so disorientated that I said I didn't want breakfast and he could go down alone if he did. He tried to kiss me, which didn't go down well considering I'd just been woken up; I needed a bit of space to come round. He wanted to go down for breakfast and once I'd come round, I realised that of course I wanted food!

I stayed in the room and washed my hair while he had breakfast. After a good long shower I was wide-awake and raring to go. I joined him and ordered my breakfast and then he went to check out. Once we were packed, he asked for another quickie, so we had one last tumble before he left me in the room. My auntie and uncle were picking me up at 11.

Peter was very easy-going, and aside from the snoring and rubbish jokes I'd enjoyed his company and he said he had mine too, and that he'd like to meet again another time.

My auntie and uncle arrived and I told them a little about my exciting couple of days. That afternoon, I was due to go to a party with them and my cousin Vickie. When we got there, I started to panic about what I would say if anyone asked me what I did for a living. My uncle's family are all laid-back and easygoing, so my cousin and aunt told me to just be honest. But my uncle wasn't sure. There was someone he thought would have a problem with my job: a guy called Nigel. Sometimes I find it really awkward; I don't want to embarrass anyone, but equally I feel just as uncomfortable if I lie about it.

My aunt had told Nigel's wife that she had a niece who worked as an escort and she'd thought it was no big deal, saying jokingly that if she was a few years younger, she'd be doing it!

I felt on edge. There were around 15 people at the party, six of whom were younger than me. The host was lovely and I started talking to her elderly mother. Silently, I prayed she wouldn't ask what I did as I hadn't decided what I was going to say. She asked if I worked in Nottingham, and I said yes, and that I was self-employed. 'Have you always lived in Bristol?' I asked, randomly changing the subject. It worked, phew!

I stuck by my cousin and spent most of the time talking with her instead of mingling. Eventually, after a short conversation with Nigel's wife, she asked what I did. As she was the one my auntie had already told (she may have suspected I was the niece, but didn't know for sure), I told her in a hushed whisper. 'Oh, fabulous – I bet that's exciting!' 'That's why I was down in Bristol at Thornbury Castle,' I explained. She said that she'd thought it was a bit extravagant of me to be staying at Thornbury for the weekend, and that explained things.

Then, saved by the bell, the food arrived – which nipped that conversation in the bud! Thankfully, we left shortly afterwards.

CHAPTER 6:

Back to Reality

I spent many hours working on the documentary that I'd been filming for some time with the friendly ladies from the TV company, but by the time I started working, I didn't have so much time to spend with them and I'd begun to lose interest. My mum and the rest of the family were interviewed about my new profession. They filmed Mum in the kitchen, saying that she was half-expecting it when I started my dancing career, but that I was selling myself short and could do much better for myself. She was also mainly concerned for my safety.

My brothers made jokes, one of them saying he hoped I wouldn't do any more magazine work as he'd be horrified to pick up a top-shelf magazine, settle down at home to enjoy it and then find his sister in there! My other brother said I had an easy job. In his eyes all I did was get paid to go out for dinner with people. If only he knew how difficult it was to keep talking and showing an interest in someone when you may find them incredibly boring.

After a month or so of working, I found the job wasn't as easy as I had first thought. I found it emotionally draining and I became quite withdrawn. I didn't have a proper social life and didn't want to talk to my friends. None of my friends had judged me because most of them knew that I was a bit eccentric. But I literally put everything into my work and found I didn't want to socialise outside of my job, so I rarely went out or did anything apart from work. It took a while for me to adapt and to find ways to deal with the emotional side of being an escort, so that the guys I met didn't take everything out of me.

This is when I realised I'd have to turn into a bit of a control freak, not with others but with myself where work was concerned, to protect my sanity and deal with my job. People know upfront what to expect from me and what I expect from them, as I make it clear from my website and reviews, so if my expectations don't match theirs then we don't meet up. If they haven't done their homework and we do meet, then we both end up disappointed.

Part of the stress was due to me living at home and having the smallest bedroom. I'd come in from overnight dates and go to bed, but be woken up by inconsiderate members of my family. I desperately needed my own place. Sharing a bathroom at home with five others was a nightmare. I'd think I had plenty of time to get myself ready, but just as I was about to get in the bath, my brother would go in, spend ages in there *and* use all the hot water. Not quite the glamorous life of a high-class escort!

Even though my mum didn't agree with my choice of profession, she was an absolute star and very supportive. If I was stressing out, often she would give me a pep-talk and get me a cup of tea, then try and calm me down and get me in the right frame of mind for work. Understandably, Mum had decided that she didn't want me living at home once my escorting became serious. When she saw the money I was earning, she suggested that I bought somewhere rather than rent. I found a place and thankfully she let me stay while I sorted out buying the apartment.

By this time I had lost interest in the TV documentary – I wasn't getting paid for it anyway. However, I made sure they got the rest of their footage. I had to go and meet the guy from the original listings site, UK Escorts, in Nottingham and although I never did a job with them and no longer wanted a listing, I had to pretend I was signing up. There was a dummy interview with the boss of the company, Colin, who clearly knew nothing about the escorting scene. I had to think of questions to ask him and my first question on camera was about safety, to which his response was, 'Carry a gun.' Funny guy! Then he wanted to stop the cameras while he found a copy of one of his brochures – the one I'd received in my welcome pack. He claimed to have written it, but he couldn't remember any of the information. It was basic, commonsense stuff, most of which I'd figured out for myself, yet he had to read up on it. Idiot! I gave him a few suggestions off the top of my head. For instance, always tell someone where you're going and be sure to get the client's full name and a contact number, etc. That wrapped up the programme and I was glad to be rid of my little entourage. The documentary was eventually broadcast in April 2001.

A solicitor I met offered to help me out once I'd found an apartment I wanted to buy. He was a great help and before long, I had moved out and was making it on my own.

Diary: March 2008

'Where be you to, Rach?' asked my regular client from Cornwall. 'I "be" in the apartment block and I can't find you. Can you come back to Reception and meet me there?' I asked.

Tom is hilarious. His accent gives me the giggles, and he doesn't mind me mimicking him. It's impossible not to. I love the 'Where be it to?' which he frequently asks about various things, and another expression I like is when he says he has 'tuth' ache, instead of toothache.

I meet Tom about half a dozen times a year. In his early fifties and single, he's a season ticket holder for Derby County and I often meet him in Derby. I've sometimes been with him to watch the football, but our regular thing is concerts. He's taken me to some amazing shows. We've seen The Eagles twice (once being last night), Christina Aguilera, Bryan Adams, Elton John, Texas (twice) and Steve Winwood, among others. We've also seen a couple of musicals.

95

I have taken on the role of finding us hotels and restaurants to go to, because he's not so much of a snob as me. It's because I don't trust him to put as much time and effort into researching as I do – we used to eat at the Harvester! I absolutely hate chain pubs – they tend to serve overpriced food that's been defrosted and microwaved, or deep-fried, bought-in food. After getting a dicky tummy one night and having to leave him in the middle of our date, it was the perfect excuse not to go to a chain pub again. So I searched the Internet, read reviews and managed to find a Chinese a short cab ride away. Now, that's where we eat when we're in Derby.

Our date last night was to see an Eagles concert at the O2 arena in London. Neither of us had been before, so I set about the task of finding a hotel and restaurant for us. My research showed that London Bridge would be a convenient area to get to from the concert, and easy for us both to get back to our train stations the next day. I trawled through reviews online and found some apartments which I thought would be ideal; we could book a two-bedroom so that we could both get a good night's sleep. He's another bad snorer! Then I asked an escort site for restaurant recommendations. I decided on one called Fish and booked us in for 5.30p.m.

When he eventually found me at Reception, we made our way up to our apartment. It was wonderfully spacious. We didn't have long as it was after 5p.m. when I arrived, and he'd only just got there himself so he didn't have any time to relax either. He changed and we went straight out.

The restaurant was a short walk from our apartment. Over dinner he asked how the twins were doing. This bit of banter was initiated by me as I refer to my boobs as 'the twins' (a saying I picked up from *The League of Gentlemen*), and now it's become a regular thing. I even sign my emails, 'love from Rach and the twins'. He is definitely a boob man and loves it if I wear low-cut tops and push-up bras, which I usually do. 'They're doing very well, thanks. They're pleased to see you after all this time,' was my reply, with a big grin. 'You've been neglecting them,' I added. 'They're looking very well,' he noted, looking at them appreciatively. We had an hour and a half before setting off for the concert, so we enjoyed a leisurely three courses before he settled the bill and we went to get a cab.

We made it just as the concert was starting. It was a fabulous evening, but by the time we'd got the boat back to London Bridge and a cab to the hotel, it was way past my bedtime.

We didn't waste any time getting naked and into bed. He told me he's been wanking over me. It turns me on to think of him sat at home, wanking over my pictures or just fantasising about me. So I asked him how many times he's done it and what he was imagining. He said he'd done it three out of every four nights. I don't have penetrative sex with Tom, nor do I give him more than a few seconds of oral because his thing is breast relief. Every time, that's all he wants to do. It turns me on too, and I love men coming on my boobs, so it suits me fine. He doesn't give me oral sex, but I don't mind – I just love having him playing with my boobs and I'll use my toy, if I want to climax. He comes very quickly, so I can barely touch his penis. Every time I touch it even gently, he has to move my hand away after a couple of strokes. So, he played with my boobs and then wanked in them as I held them together for him.

In the morning I got into bed with him and snuggled up. He lay there, not moving at all or initiating anything, even though I'd taken my top off. He was still dozing. I lay there for about 15 minutes or so before getting up and grabbing a shower. Then I cooked us eggs and toast for breakfast before leaving him in the apartment to go and get my train.

CHAPTER 7:

A-levels – a Lot to Learn

You wouldn't think there could be so many complicated terms involved in the sex business! It took me ages to figure out what all the terminology meant. I was asked if I offered A-levels, which I thought was a schoolgirl fantasy thing, and replied that I hadn't got A-levels, but I did have GCSEs. I never heard back from him! Later, I found out that 'A-levels' meant anal sex – I felt really stupid. 'O-levels' is oral sex. I hadn't even heard of London being called 'the Big Smoke', as I hadn't been there since I was about 13 or 14. When someone asked if I could go to the Big Smoke, I wondered what on earth he was talking about.

I used to go to the library to check my emails, but as the computers were in the children's section this wasn't ideal given the nature of some of my correspondence. I remember it was once full of kids and mums and I happened to open an email attachment. A guy had sent me a close-up photo of his private parts. I was horrified as the huge picture gradually downloaded on the screen. Not knowing anything about computers, I didn't know how to stop it – it was so embarrassing, trying to hide it from everyone in there.

When I think back to that time, I realise I was very naïve. I didn't know what to wear for my dates – I was still wearing my chunky platforms and clubbing clothes. As I didn't know any escorts, everything I learnt I had to find out for myself. There was one guy from my early days that I remember, who was a solicitor, and I had asked him if he would like me to dress casually or smartly. He replied smartly, as he'd be wearing his suit from work. My idea of 'smart' was this little ensemble: snake-print tight PVC hipsters, a pair of black platform sandals, a child-sized grey cardigan that I had no chance of buttoning up, tied in a knot at the front to show a little bit of cleavage, a bright pink-and-purple bra and a pink fluffy Barbie bag. Oh, how I cringe now! Fortunately, he was very open-minded and found it amusing. I stuck out like a sore thumb in that posh hotel in Birmingham; we looked so out-of-place together.

God knows how, but I still managed to get some very professional regulars (bankers, accountants and solicitors), who I saw monthly for overnights and who all took me out for dinner in public.

Last year I saw someone who confessed that he'd seen me a few years before, when I had just started out. I asked him why he hadn't wanted to see me again and he said it was because – and I remember this outfit so clearly – I had worn a leather-look mini with a skimpy top and platform dancing stilettos to go out to dinner! I'm not sure why I did that because I'd usually wear trousers – it's the only time I've been out in a mini for work. He didn't have the guts to say anything at the time, but he was extremely embarrassed, going to the top London restaurant that we ate in. I remember the room was long and narrow, and our table was right at the back, so we had to walk past everyone. When I asked why he'd booked me again, he said he'd seen me recently on a date and noticed that I now dress more discreetly.

I remember one date I had with my solicitor friend; he decided to surprise me and take me to London. We drove down together and he told me that he had arranged for us to go on a limousine ride around London, with champagne, and then to see the musical *Chicago*. I was so excited! We had a couple of drinks at the hotel before jumping in the limo. I had never been inside one before and couldn't believe I was being paid to be in one and to be taken to the theatre. After sharing a bottle of champagne on an empty stomach, I was actually quite drunk. I told him I needed to get some food, so we stopped at a takeaway and I ran in and got pizza. I didn't really like the pizza and it was rather cold, so I only had one piece.

The show was amazing, but it was all a bit of a blur. I had no idea what was going on because I was very tipsy. Back at the hotel I passed out, and in the morning I had a steaming hangover. He was chuckling to himself because he asked me how I felt, and I just muttered with half-opened, puffy eyes, 'I feel like shit!' He was convinced I just needed feeding, so we had a big banquet sent up to the room. However, after a few mouthfuls I was dashing to the loo to be sick. It was awful and very embarrassing. I did get paid, but my date had no sex at all that meeting! But people pay for my time, not sex. I did feel guilty, but I knew I would make it up to him the next time. After all, it was partly his fault for not feeding me before the show!

These are the kind of mistakes I have learnt from. Now, I would never drink that much on an empty stomach and I check when and where we will eat. I also ask what the gentleman meeting me is going to wear for our date, and I find out whether there's a dress code for wherever we're going.

Diary: December 2008

I stood in the never-ending queue, shivering with cold, as the wind and rain blew through the open doorway where we were all waiting for taxis. It took a while for the penny to drop, but I soon realised why so many people with cases were waiting there. They had obviously come off the Eurostar at St Pancras, which had just opened. It was smack-bang in the middle of rush hour. 'Great,' I thought, 'I'm going to be late, which means I'll feel obliged to stay late on my date.'

Fortunately the queue went down very quickly, the traffic wasn't too bad and, surprisingly, I got to my destination a little earlier than 6p.m. As I confidently breezed through, trying to locate the lifts, I did a quick scan of the hotel. I walked straight past the lifts before realising my mistake and backtracking. This was the perfect hotel layout – I didn't have to walk past Reception; I just walked through the front door and the lifts were there on my right.

As an escort I have to look like I know where I'm going, and be confident and discreet. I never wear tarty or revealing clothes on my dates. As I'm not checking in, I don't want to be questioned by hotel staff. Some London hotels are on the lookout for escorts, and have turned ladies away; others turn a blind eye.

Even though we would be eating at a Michelin-starred restaurant, I'd been asked to wear jeans. When my overweight American date opened the door in a pair of tatty grey jogging bottoms and a New York T-shirt pebble-dashed with toothpaste, my heart sank. Surely he couldn't seriously be thinking of going out like that?

The room was large and spacious, and the bed was huge, I was pleased to note. It would have been awful to share a smaller bed with him because of his sheer size. I don't mind big men at all, though, because for me it really is about people's personality: looks are only a bonus. We sat on the sofa and he poured us both glasses of champagne. It transpired he was single, and I guessed he was in his fifties (thanks to his comb-over hairstyle, where all the hair on one side was long enough to be draped from one side of his head, across the bald patch in the middle to the other side). He worked as an accountant. He'd made our dinner reservation for 7.30p.m., and there was no way I'd be able to polish off half a bottle of champagne before eating. I'd be hammered! So I sipped mine while he had two large glasses. Please don't let him get pissed, I silently prayed.

When guys get nervous they sometimes drink too much – and then they can't get it up, and they snore like a trooper! I counted my fee, £1,000, and thanked him before discreetly putting it in my bag. Once that bit is out of the way, I can relax and enjoy the evening. He seemed surprised that I had turned up, and said he didn't think I would. Apparently he'd booked another lady earlier in the week and she had left after their expensive dinner, giving him half the money back and saying that they didn't get along. This sounded an odd thing for her to have done, especially as he seemed pleasant enough. She was well-known and had good feedback on the escort review sites (where our looks and performance are rated), but I didn't really know what to say because it wouldn't have been fair to pass judgement without hearing her side of the story.

He'd kindly bought me some lingerie as a gift. It's always a pleasant surprise to get presents – they're not expected, but they're always appreciated. When he said we'd be walking to the restaurant, I was a bit put out. I don't mind walking short distances, but it was so cold and rainy that I was dreading going outside. I asked if he had a jacket I could borrow. He said he did, but that it wasn't cold, and I corrected him by saying that just because he wasn't cold, it didn't mean others wouldn't be.

He began to argue with me and it got my back up – some people are so self-obsessed. He wasn't getting the message, so I cheekily told him I didn't have any fat to keep me warm, and that if I was cold on the way there, I'd be getting a cab back on my own. You tend to find this with single men; they aren't used to thinking about other people. I call it SMS – Single Man Syndrome. He told me I wouldn't be cold in his jacket, and I said he had no way of knowing how I might feel. I also told him he didn't seem to care about my comfort, but he insisted he was a gentleman. I said he wasn't being very gentlemanly by expecting me to walk just because he liked walking and wasn't cold. This little scenario did make me wonder if I too would be running off after dinner; I was finding him very difficult to get along with.

Fortunately he changed into a shirt and jeans, and put on a long overcoat for dinner. I put on his old casual, burnt orange coat, which drowned me. He said it suited me… Hmm! Outside, he noticed that it was raining, so he decided he wanted to get a cab. I could have told him it was raining! I debated whether to take his jacket back upstairs, but decided there was no point, especially as he thought I looked so good in it.

In the restaurant we both ordered fish starters, and then I had lamb while he ordered sole. He ended up with white bits of fish all over his face, and I was horrified. I had to keep asking him to wipe his face with his napkin, but as there was so much fish on the napkin, he ended up moving it around his face rather than removing it. How on earth could he not realise his face was covered with fish? Then I thought back to the toothpaste on the T-shirt and thought, probably quite easily! Clearly, he was oblivious to any mess he made.

It was bizarre and quite embarrassing, especially as we were surrounded by other diners. I have noticed that men who live on their own often have zero table manners. He spent ages picking at his teeth, because he had a fish bone stuck between them. Eager to get him to stop picking, I called the waiter, who brought over some toothpicks. He had de-boned the fish, but obviously missed all the small bones, so he sat there with his face covered in fish, picking bones out of his mouth. I couldn't disguise the look of disgust on my face, yet he seemed oblivious. I wonder if the other escort was so repulsed by his eating habits that this was the reason she had taken off without going to bed with him.

We had a twenty-minute breather before ordering desserts. He had the ice cream and I had the cheese, and all in all, we were at the restaurant for a good three hours. Socialising is the main part of my job – I love to eat at quality restaurants, so if we can get to know one another over dinner in a fine restaurant then I'm more than happy. We headed back to the hotel around 11p.m. and I changed into one of the lingerie sets he had bought me. The bra was a size too small, so I was popping out, but I didn't think he'd mind.

I lay beside him and we French-kissed. We spent a while caressing each other – I was worried he'd be an eager beaver, but thankfully he wasn't. Eventually he slid his boxers off and helped me out of my lingerie. I stroked his penis and down his thighs and I could feel him harden with my touch. At one point I thought he would just fall asleep. He lay there, with his eyes closed, on the bed. I then just rested beside him because I wasn't sure if he wanted to sleep as he wasn't touching me. I'm not paid to entertain sexually – whatever goes on in the bedroom is about two-way enjoyment, so the more clients put into it, the more they get out of it.

I'm always nervous about the first time with a client as I don't know what to expect – whether he'll be one that can hold an erection and take forever to come, or one that comes easily with minimal effort. Fortunately, he was the latter. Obviously, if it's someone who comes quickly, I try to drag out the foreplay so that his fun can last longer. If they take forever, it's extremely hard work and I want to get down to business with less foreplay.

After cuddling for a while, he eventually went down on me and I squirmed with pleasure (when the pressure was just right), and a little bit of discomfort (when he was too firm). He did this for a few minutes, before popping his head up to let me know he was done down there. I took the hint and he lay on his back while I took him in my mouth; I alternated sucking him and using my hands. Although he had said that he wanted to be inside me, it wasn't long before I could feel him start to shudder. He didn't seem to want me to stop, so I carried on and pulled away just in time as he ejaculated all over my hand and both our bodies. I remember trying to keep the gap between our bodies closed so that none of it would drip onto the side of the bed I'd be sleeping on, but unfortunately it did. He got up and fetched a wet flannel and a towel for us to try and clean up the mess.

We both settled to go to sleep at about 12.30a.m. After a good lie-in, I stirred. He was still fast asleep, so I crept silently to the loo, and then got back in bed with him and snuggled up. Big men are far more comfortable to snuggle with than skinny ones. As I don't sleep cuddled up (I like my own space when I sleep), I always have a cuddle in the morning. He put his arm around me, and after a few minutes I decided to go down on him and get the morning session going. But he didn't seem to be responding and said he wasn't usually a morning person. So we snuggled and dozed for another hour. He'd said he didn't normally eat in the morning and I doubted he would offer me anything, so I decided to be assertive and said I was calling down to order breakfast.

I stayed longer than I would have normally, but we were dozing and I was very relaxed. I left at about 11.30a.m. and wished him well for the rest of his trip. Despite the walking issue and the fish-face problem, it was a pleasant date and I hope he'll let me know next time he's in the country.

CHAPTER 8:

Boyfriend Number
One – Kenny

I 'd been working for about a year when I met Kenny, who was to be my first boyfriend since becoming an escort. I hadn't seen anyone outside of work and getting a boyfriend was the last thing on my mind; I just figured that as soon as guys found out what I did, they wouldn't be interested in me, and I didn't want to lie and then be in a relationship based on deceit. That's what my work is, as a lot of the guys I see are married! So, I knew I would have to be honest with people in my personal life, and therefore I was prepared to be single.

Boyfriends are not my forte. In fact, it's sad to admit that I have never had a decent long-term relationship where I can say that I've been truly happy, even before my escorting. I always pick the wrong guys! As my work is in effect a series of one-night stands, they don't interest me in my personal life. I want sex outside work to mean something and to be with someone special. I don't consciously switch off with my work; I don't need to. I don't have to stop myself falling for these guys, it just doesn't happen.

I can't wait to be a mum and a wife, and spend the rest of my life with one person. I don't get any sort of kick from sleeping with strangers anymore; I just accept it as a small part of my job. I love kids, and people say I'd make a great mum. I hope to have a big family, but I'm not focusing on trying to find the man of my dreams at the moment because I really want to be successful at something else before I settle down. I'd like to meet my life partner when I've closed the escorting chapter of my life, and hopefully I'll meet someone open-minded enough not to hold my past against me. I'm very open and honest, so surely that has to count for something?

Kenny was a couple of years older than me and lived in Sheffield. I was clubbing with my sister in Chesterfield when I first spotted him – he was mixed race, about my height, and very good-looking. He was also a very cool dancer and I was instantly attracted. We caught each other's eye on the dance floor and started bumping and grinding together. After a few dances I asked him if he wanted a drink, and bought us both bottles of water. I suppose in retrospect the warning signs were there: he really should have offered *me* a drink first. He asked me what I did for a living, and I told him straight out. Then he said that he didn't have a problem with it because it was actually something that he had always wanted to do, and he was quite intrigued. We hit it off straightaway and started going out, but Kenny wanted an easy life, doing as little as possible while sponging off me. I was stupid not to see it at the time.

One might think that as an escort, meeting numerous unfaithful guys, I might not trust men, but I trusted all three of the guys I have been out with while escorting. I knew that I was keeping them happy in the bedroom department and I'm naturally affectionate. More often, it's when women don't look after their men, physically and emotionally, that they cheat.

My brothers will never forget one of the first times they met Kenny. I was moving into my apartment in Nottingham and he came to my mum's to help me with my stuff, but he just sat there while my brothers and I carried everything to the car and packed it. He didn't lift a finger to help! I can honestly say he's the tightest person I have ever had the misfortune to meet – he's so mean that he even told me he starved himself to shrink his stomach so he didn't have to spend much money on food! Also, he never bought more than a couple of drinks when he went out, even without me. At first I found it attractive that he wasn't one for going out and getting drunk, but then I realised it was because he was tight.

It seemed that being an escort *was* going to get in the way of our relationship, but not in the way you might think. He didn't have a problem with me being with other men, because he knew I would be coming back to him, but he seemed to think that I had the money to pay for everything! In the year and a half that we went out together, he bought me one meal and maybe a couple of drinks. I bought him a mobile phone and when he moved house, he didn't let me have his landline number. He'd withhold his number, call me, hang up before I answered and then expect me to call him back on his mobile! He had a well-paid job, but always claimed not to have any money – I suspect he was saving a small fortune going out with me, so he probably had a huge savings account. What a complete mug I was!

Kenny also had a massive chip on his shoulder and was harbouring a lot of hatred and resentment, mainly for his parents, to whom he hadn't spoken in years. Then one Christmas, he became aggressive. I had driven to see him in Sheffield on Christmas Eve, and when I got to the house he shared, he wasn't even in. For over an hour I waited for him and when he waltzed in, needless to say I wasn't happy as I could have spent more time with my family. He blew up and started pushing me around. Then he tried to physically stop me from leaving, and threw my keys out of his window into the dark.

I believe his behaviour stemmed from the fact that I'd received some compensation money because of problems with my apartment, and I'd decided to take my sister away to Orlando. He was so pissed off – for some bizarre reason he believed that I should have paid for him to have a free holiday. After that night, he was asked to leave the house by the couple he lived with, but I still didn't dump him. I think I'd got used to being with someone, and couldn't bear the thought of being on my own again. Maybe because I didn't think many other guys would go out with an escort, I thought I ought to make do with him… or perhaps I didn't feel I deserved any better. It seemed that whenever I had a boyfriend, I became weak, and I hated myself for it. At work I was confident, but clearly in my personal life I wasn't, or I wouldn't have put up with Kenny for a year and a half!

Then he was made redundant and had to move out of his flat. After complaining that he'd be homeless, I reluctantly said that he could move in with me. I didn't want him to because I didn't feel the time was right and I wasn't in love with him, but I thought that as his girlfriend I should help him out. So, he sat at home while I went out to work.

I know he never had a problem with my job because although we argued a lot, my work was never mentioned. I think he thought he'd hit the jackpot: an attractive woman who was willing to look after him. It was just like my relationship with James. Even though Kenny was given redundancy pay, he never offered me any cash for putting him up, saying he had to make it last. Thinking about it, he must have been getting dole money as well, but he never mentioned that to me. On my birthday I gave him money so that he could come out with me and my friends: he bought one drink, and pocketed the rest of the cash! He had absolutely no shame and couldn't see he was doing anything wrong.

I was determined he was going to pay his way, so every now and then I used to ask him to clean and to organise things on the computer for my work. He made a real fuss about the cleaning, and made no effort to do anything at all around the house. Once, I explained a few things I wanted him to do on my computer. He then came to me with a bit of paper, saying if I wanted A and B doing, it would cost me £250, and if I wanted A, B and C doing, it would be £350. I couldn't believe my ears. Of course, I should have thrown him out there and then, but I didn't. I was fuming and said if he wanted to start charging me for what he did for a living, I would make him pay for what I did for a living! For 150 overnights, say, his bill would be £120,000. I managed to put up with him for about two months before I asked him to move out.

I think being with Kenny made me more aware of people taking the piss. Now, I'm very conscious of it. I'm always aware of those who expect me to buy drinks for them, and of people who avoid buying rounds, are slow reaching for their purse or wallet, or who make comments about not being able to afford to go out when they actually go out more than me *and* have more holidays. It irritates the hell out of me. I'm naturally a very generous person, but I don't let people take advantage of it.

I'll never forget getting back in touch with one of my ex-best friends from school, a few years ago. I drove all the way over to Chesterfield to see her, and she'd forgotten I was visiting. I was fuming – I can't stand it when people waste my time. So, I had a 60-mile round trip for nothing. She rang me to apologise, and after about ten minutes said, 'Anyway, I'd better go – we can't *all* afford to be chatting on the phone for hours.' I knew then that it was unlikely we'd rekindle our friendship.

I also feel that one of my close friends, Hannah, doesn't understand about my work and my life. She lives in a bedsit, doesn't drive and works a 9–5. Hannah hasn't a clue about responsibilities, because she doesn't have any. She goes out all the time and lives for the moment, which is fine, but as I don't know how much I will earn from week to week and have a car, house and business to run, I simply cannot do that. She thinks

I'm loaded when I've had a couple of busy weeks with work, because of my high rates, but what I feel she doesn't understand (even though she claims to) is that I don't have that sort of regular work all the time, yet I still have the same high outgoings every month. I spend a fortune on my website and advertising, then there's my mortgage and other essentials, and I do pay tax, so it's not like every penny goes in my pocket. I have to make sure I always have emergency money saved for when I have a dry month.

Hannah also knows someone who works for an agency, and she probably thinks we earn the same amount. Girls working for agencies don't have to pay anything for advertising, and their time is only taken up with their work. They don't have to put any time or effort into screening clients, or sorting out advertising, or maintaining websites; they give the agency their photos and just wait for the jobs to roll in. Usually they don't pay tax either, so all the money's in their back pockets; they probably earn more money than me and use less of their time.

Our priorities are different. Yes, I may spend £200 on a pair of shoes sometimes, but I don't go out at all during the week and rarely socialise at weekends. Hannah will spend £200 a week on going out. She does more socially than I do, and she actually has more disposable income than me, but I know she thinks I'm loaded. I love her dearly, and we have such great fun when we are together, but I just wish she was more understanding about my work situation and my responsibilities.

I feel very uncomfortable when friends want to see my website because they just see the high rates and think, 'wow!' They have no idea how much work I get, or how much disposable income I'm left with at the end of the month. People have a false impression – I'm not rolling in money. I do get to visit spectacular restaurants, eat incredible food and see stunning sights, but someone else is always paying, not me.

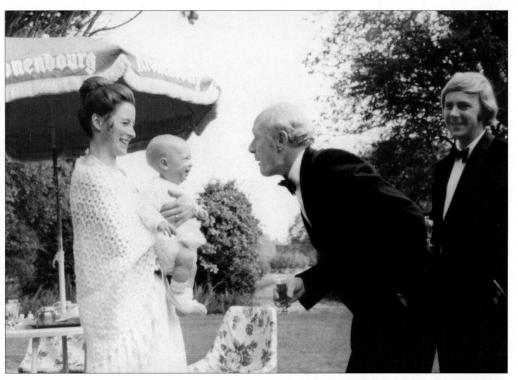

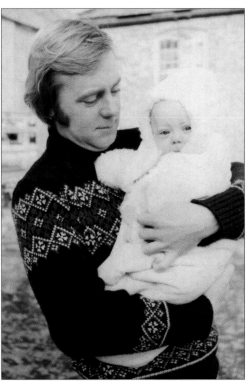

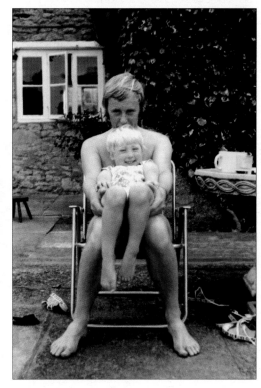

Above: Me with my beautiful mum.

Below left: Here I am all snuggled and warm on my Granny's farm.

Below right: Daddy's girl.

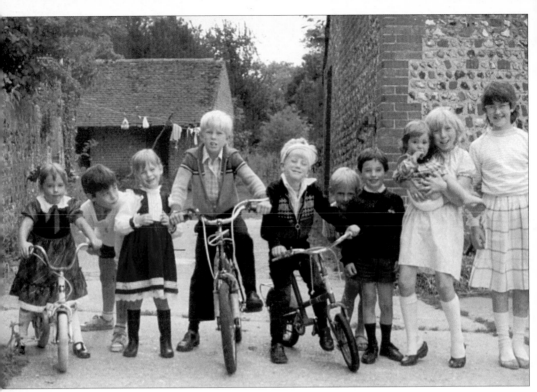

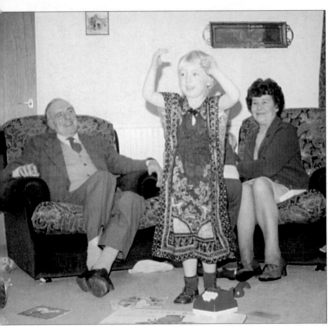

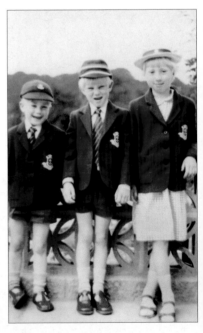

Above: Here's all the farm crew! We still have great, legendary parties with our cousins on my uncle's farm.

Below left: Impressing the family with one of my grandma's dance routines. She brought the dress back from one of her holidays.

Below right: Under the brown and gold – our hideous convent uniforms and my dodgy hair. We all had the same haircut!

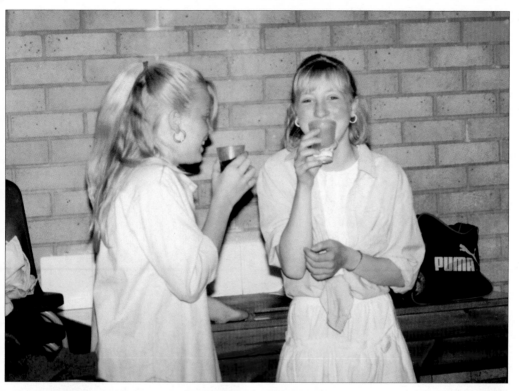

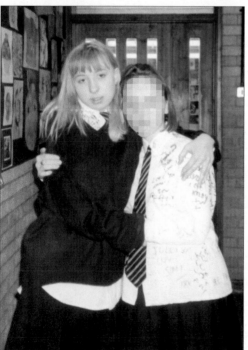

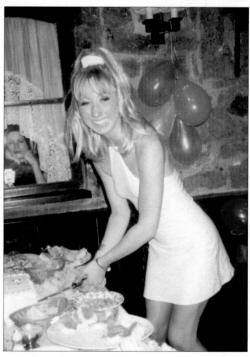

Above: Aged 13 at a secondary school disco, wearing my dad's shirt.
I always pinched his clothes!

Below left: Football face! This was my last day at school.

Below right: My 21st. I look like a drag queen! Ha!

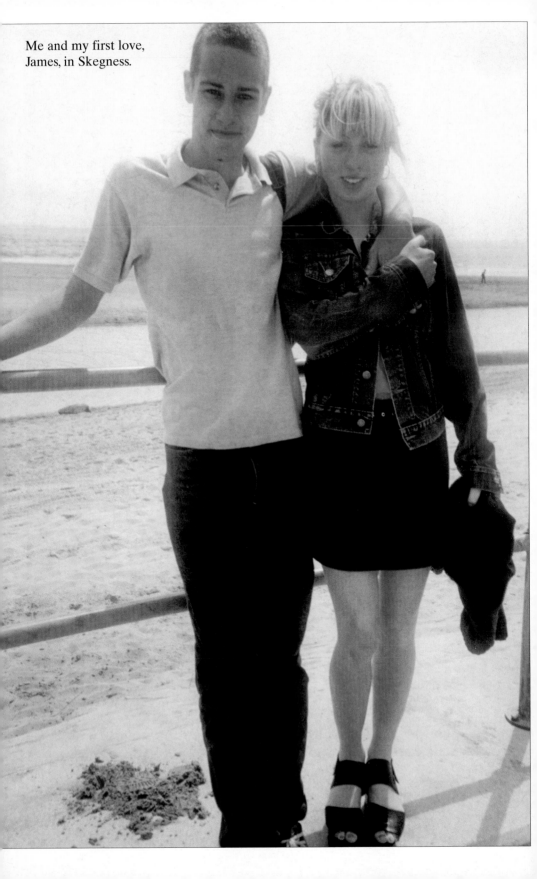

Me and my first love,
James, in Skegness.

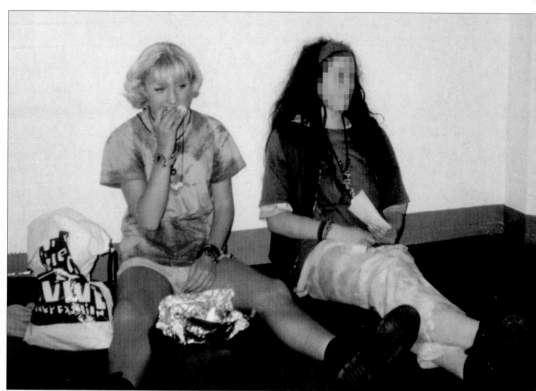

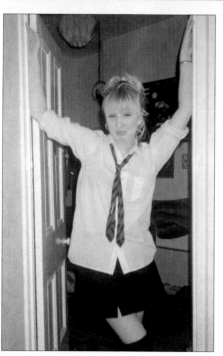
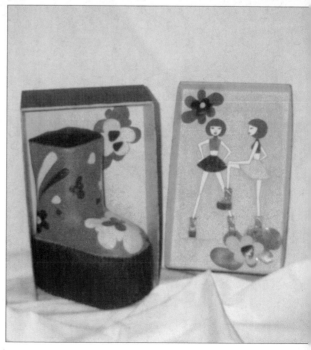

Above: Here I am as a glammed-up hippy aged 17, stuffing my face with a sandwich! Nice.

Below left: Aged 18, in my fave college outfit. So risqué!

Below right: My platform welly for a Shelly's shoe design competition. They missed out on a young budding designer whose designs were way ahead of her time!

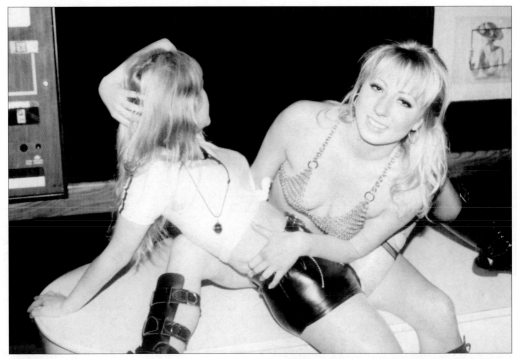

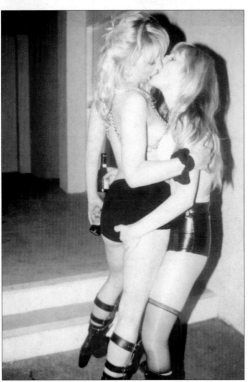
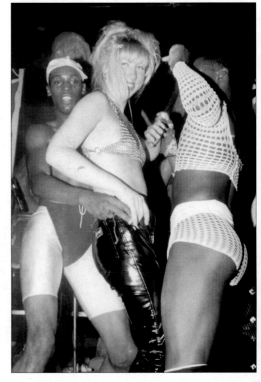

Above: Tara and me in the Hollywood bar posing at Xanadu's, Chez Vegas!

Below left: Misbehaving in the back room of Xanadu's.

Below right: I got pulled onto the stage by two hunky black men (nice bum on the right!) on one of Jon's photography nights out.

All © Jon Edgington

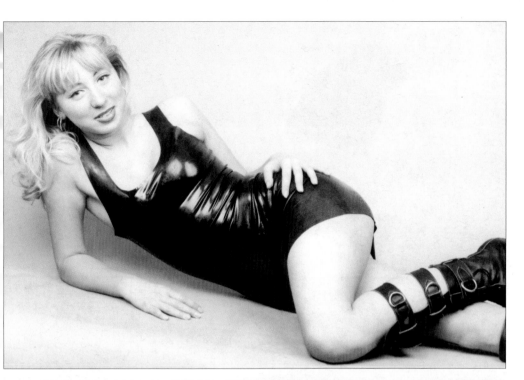

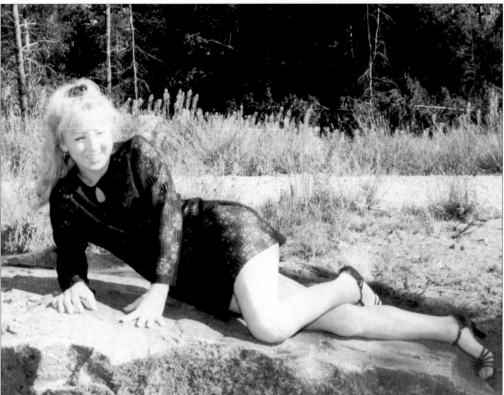

Above: An early glamour shoot in one of my favourite outfits.

Below: My first ever glamour shoot aged 18, with my favourite see-through dress. I was not and still am not a natural model... can you tell?

© *Jon Edgington*

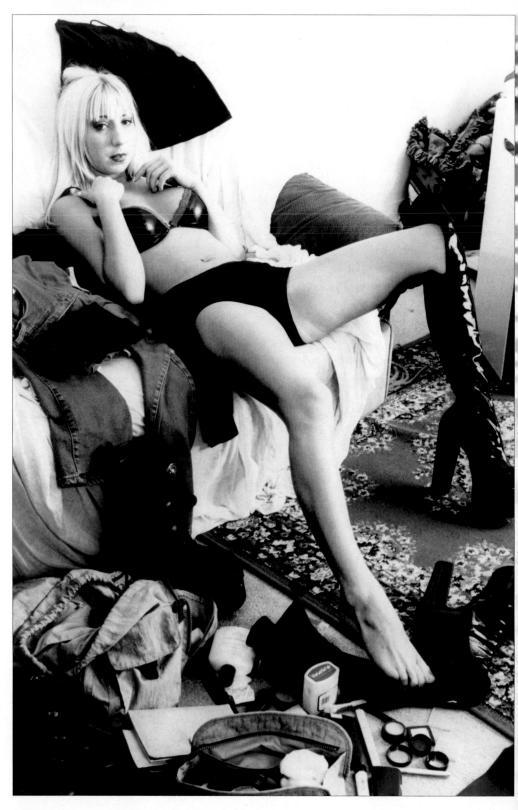

This was pretty much how I would go out. It took me a while to learn that less is more!

Diary: February 2008

'I'm sorry, I'm looking for a non-English girl,' was the email response I had when I replied to an advert a guy had placed on the escort site Captain 69, looking for someone to take to Cirque du Soleil at London's Royal Albert Hall. Charming, I thought. Why would someone specifically want a non-English escort? Perhaps they're cheaper, or maybe if they don't speak much English, they won't waste too much time with conversation! I get the feeling a lot of the Eastern European escorts aren't as assertive as some of the English girls like me, so they can be taken advantage of.

It was the last weekend of the show's run, and I was desperate to go. I remembered Charly, a young 24-year-old virgin that I had met a couple of years ago (no, I didn't pop his cherry by the way!). When I last saw him, he was working in a bar. He comes from a rich family, but I didn't get the impression that he got handouts, so he must have paid for our last date himself, which cost him a fortune. It was a 24-hour date and we stayed at Claridge's.

Charly's a very nervous person and I suppose he's a bit geeky. Although he's a really sweet guy, I imagine he struggles socially. He's average height, a little overweight with dark, wiry ginger hair. We'd been liaising about a meeting since December and I hadn't heard from him for a few weeks. As it was now mid-February, I decided to be assertive and email him asking about a date, suggesting we might go to the Cirque du Soleil show. I sent him links so that he could see if it was something he'd like.

I was pleasantly surprised when he got back to me promptly and was very keen on the idea, saying he'd heard about the show and wanted to go. If I can tie in things that I really want to see with getting paid to work, it's a bonus! He bought us matinee tickets and to fit with his plans, I said I'd come to London for 2p.m. and leave at 9p.m.: an extended dinner date.

In the hotel room he gave me my envelope, and when I counted the notes I saw he'd paid me £20 extra. I told him it was a good job I checked it and gave him a note back. We caught a cab, and I noticed his face was literally dripping with sweat – I think it was nerves. He spoke about a girlfriend that he'd had for a couple of weeks, but I could tell that he was still a virgin.

We arrived with about ten minutes to spare enough time to get the tickets, a drink and settle into our seats. With six others, we were in one of the many lines of boxes (like The Muppet Show, with red curtains). The show was fantastic! Awkwardly, he tried to put his arm around me, but decided to remove it after a couple of minutes. I like to be discreet, especially as I do get recognised sometimes, so although I consider myself naturally very affectionate and tactile, I'm not so much in public.

While walking around afterwards looking for a restaurant, I recognised the glass porch to the Baglioni, a 5-star hotel in Kensington with a fabulous Italian restaurant inside, so we decided to eat there. We ordered aperitifs and perused the menu. A starter of lobster linguine was double the price of all the others, at £25! But when he ordered it, I decided to do the same. The food was fantastic. We left the restaurant with an hour and a half to spare and thankfully got a cab straightaway.

Back in the room I said I'd run a bath. We had arranged this by email before the date, because last time he hadn't told me he was a virgin and the bedroom side of things was a bit of a disaster — I didn't know what he wanted or expected. So, this time, we communicated and arranged that we'd bathe together to relax and get us in the mood, and then we'd take things slowly and play it by ear. I ran the bath and lit candles. We only had an hour, so there wasn't as much time to relax as I would have liked. We got into the bath and I put my legs over his and leant in to kiss him. His body was rigid and he tried to hold me into a kiss by clamping his arm and hand around my back and head. Gently, I pushed him off and told him to relax — it's a big turn-off for me to be clamped! I know it was nerves, but I needed to tell him because if he does that with other women, they won't like it and probably won't have the guts to tell him.

But I knew it was just because he was nervous and excited. As he cupped my breasts, he was trembling and tried very hard to relax with his kissing. He complimented my body and I reached through the water to grab his penis. Though he wasn't hard, with some gentle pulling he stiffened in my grasp. I wanted him to enjoy our time as much as possible, so I suggested we moved to the bed to get more comfy.

I said I always liked to moisturise after bathing and asked if he'd like to rub in some oil. He was more than happy to oblige, and spent a while massaging it in until he lingered on my breasts before taking them in his mouth in turn. He seemed happy to stay there for most of the time we had left, while I masturbated him. My hand was sticky with pre-come, his whole body dripping with sweat. I could tell he wouldn't come in the time we had left.

Conscious of time, I asked what he'd like me to do to him and reminded him that we didn't have long. He said he was happy pleasuring me! I was actually incredibly turned on as he sucked my breasts and played with his fingers down below, and I could feel myself become dripping wet. He asked if he could go down on me and spent a few minutes down there before moving back up to my breasts. At this point, I decided that I really couldn't leave without having an orgasm so I reached for my toy and brought myself very quickly to a climax.

There wasn't time to really relax and cuddle afterwards, unfortunately, and I didn't want to miss my train, so I gathered my belongings and left, thanking him for a lovely day and evening. He said he may be moving to America, so I'm not sure we'll meet again.

CHAPTER 9:

Bye, Bye, Barbie!

W hen I realised that I was building up a good reputation for myself, I knew I had to set out on my own. I didn't want to be known only through the listing site. Also, I realised that Ade could pull the plug on my business at any time if he decided to take the site down, and I didn't want to rely on anyone else. So I decided to change my name, my image, and set up my own website.

My solicitor friend knew me as both Beki and Barbie, and used to call me 'Miss B', so when I decided to change my name I hastily opted for Miss B. With hindsight, although original, it's a ridiculous name, and some said it suggested I was a dominatrix. But once I'd changed it, I thought I was stuck with it because I didn't want to confuse people – in my short time as an escort I had built a good reputation and needed clients to be able to find me. The girls who mess people around are always changing their names so they can't be traced and bad reviews aren't linked with them. As all my reviews for overnight dates were very positive, I didn't want to risk changing my name again, so Miss B, or 'B', as I preferred to be called, became my new working name.

An 18-year-old lad who lived near my mum said he would design a website for me. I couldn't visualise what I wanted and it was hard to know if he would be able to create something I would be happy with – the only websites he had done were for mechanics and accountants! I only knew what I didn't want: a cheap, tacky site that used a standard template. So, I asked him to create a clean, unfussy site, which was classy, easy to navigate and also quick to download, original and eye-catching.

I gave him a CD with some photos on it, and waited to see what he came up with. He created a front page for me and I was thrilled with what he had put together. I had never seen anything like it: he had used a photo of me in a black mini-dress, sitting on a blue blow-up chair. It was an eye-catching photo because of the colours, and as he had cut it out and put it on a white background, it really stood out. On the left was a series of white boxes, which he said would be the menu. Scrolled over, they became pink.

It was perfect, so I started writing all the text for my site. My website cost £700. I could have had one designed for a couple of hundred pounds but I wanted something different and the website Justin created for me was ideal. These days, I still get complimented on my site and often get told it's one of the best escort sites around. Most people can tell I take pride in my business by seeing the work that goes into my site. Even though I've had a number of web designers, until recently the layout has stayed the same. However, it's constantly evolving as I think of new ideas. Once my site was designed, I had it linked to my profile on an escorts' website and researched different websites on which to advertise.

It was also time to change my image. I thought perhaps I'd better dress a bit more subtly, and so I went out and bought my first-ever knee-length skirt. Shortly afterwards, I purchased my first pair of expensive shoes, black strappy sandals from Gina – they cost me £215. I took on a whole new image. I wanted to be ladylike, discreet and look classy. Gradually I built my wardrobe up to include smart trousers and knee-length pencil skirts, with feminine, sexy blouses and tops. I also started wearing dresses; I wanted to look sophisticated, elegant and sexy without showing much flesh. I didn't want to wear anything tarty that made me look like an escort. I'd take short skirts for the bedroom, but I'd never go out to work in one.

I had a number of positive reviews from my overnight dates on the review site Punternet, and these would generate business for me. I also became a member on the review site Captain 69, and started to receive glowing reviews on there too. So, people got to know me as an independent escort through my website rather than through the listings site I was on. On a usual day I spend most of my time on the Internet. I'm sure many people imagine an escort has nothing to do in the day and sits on her backside, dolled up, watching daytime TV and waiting for the phone to ring, but when I'm not out on a job, I'm spending hours trying to get work. I would say I spend about six to eight hours per day on the Internet – that's the hours of a full-time job, even before I actually go out on any dates!

My time is spent answering emails, checking new reviews on the Captain 69 site, checking the members' message board, and replying to anything of interest on the forum, where site users can chat to each other. I have got work before thanks to things I've said on the forum. I find writing very difficult, so it takes me a long time to think of what to say and how to say it. So, after I add to a thread, I monitor it and see if anyone replies directly to anything I say, or if there's someone that I can reply to. I often send people a private message rather than adding to the thread – it's more personal and it starts a bit of conversation that might lead to a date.

I don't appeal to the majority of people on the forums

because I'm very outspoken. People either love or hate me for it, but I simply couldn't be false, like many ladies are, just to get more work. I can be fun, but if I disagree or feel strongly about serious issues, I'll say so. You get a lot of people deliberately winding others up just to get a reaction, but I never take the bait if I think someone's doing that. Because of my strong views, a lot of people think I'm stuck-up, but I'm not. I just know I expect to be treated with respect, and there are many guys who don't respect women in my profession. I'm also told that I'm unique in my views on my work. I guess I am, but I'm successful and I know many people respect the way I run my business, and the person I am.

If possible I like to choose the hotel for my dates (it's in my best interest; I'm going there too), so I spend a lot of time checking accommodation and emailing people about potential hotels or reading reviews online before I make any recommendations. Checking my transport options is also very time consuming, and I always offer to look into restaurants and read reviews, so I can make sure I eat somewhere decent on my dates. Most guys don't have the time to do any research, so I know they appreciate me taking the time to do it for them. I treat any enquiries about trips abroad seriously, but sometimes I put a lot of time into checking flights and other information and then they don't come to fruition. It can be frustrating, but it's worth it for those that do work out.

The reason I have to put all this time in is because when someone asks me how much it would cost for me to visit New York for two nights I can't just give them my usual two-night rate. With all the travelling, it could end up being more like three nights. I don't charge for travelling time within the UK, but if I'm going abroad, I have to take travel into consideration. If I have to fly from London in the early morning, I'll probably go down the night before. Travelling can exhaust me, so I make it as quick and easy as possible so that I can be at my best when I arrive, and I look at all the available flights before I quote my rate.

I also advertise on a website called Northern Angels, which has a forum and a chat room. I monitor the reviews on this site, and I also frequent the forum – which is more light-hearted than the one on Captain 69. Topics have ranged from breaking wind to embarrassing things you do when you get the giggles, ogling girls' new photos and other fun stuff. There are some really lovely people on these sites, but also some idiots. The NA guys tend not to like my outspoken personality and members tend to go for either new girls or young girls, who are more easily pleased and will often put up with anything. Sometimes, I get the feeling that many guys don't like to see girls with a brain and their own opinion.

Some of the girls on there are not very bright and the guys seem to like that. This observation is based on the stupid, careless and often dangerous situations they get themselves into, which they then discuss on the 'girls' board' – a forum that's only supposed to be visible to Northern Angels girls. Some silly girls give guys access to it, though, which causes all sorts of problems. Guys don't like my assertive 'put-up-with-no-shit' attitude. There are only a few people on the site who will really stand up to someone when they disagree with them, but I have no hesitation in saying what I think. Often, I get private emails thanking me for standing up to someone or praising me for speaking my mind, but unfortunately those same people don't want to publicise that they agree with me, which is a shame.

Sometimes the escort world has its problems. For example, there are guys who will only see one lady. I understand why they do this, and I do appreciate a certain amount of loyalty, but things may get confusing because it can seem like a real relationship to the guy. Some girls also get jealous and don't want their guys to see anyone else, which further confuses the guys into thinking they are in a real relationship. They honestly feel like they've cheated on their regular escort if they see another one!

I'm always interested in what other girls my guys have seen, but I don't appreciate it when they go on and on about all the girls they see. It's not about being jealous, it's respect. Sometimes, I'll be on a date with a guy and all he'll talk about is another escort. I just think it's a bit rude... imagine if I talked about my favourite clients? But I would rather my regulars saw other ladies now and then if it stops them getting too attached to me.

There are quite a few guys who become totally delusional, and escort sites like NA become their whole life. Some single guys become so absorbed in the escort world that I don't think they even try to find a real girlfriend. In fact, they think they have many girlfriends, but they are all paid escorts. I think seeing escorts has unrealistically raised the standards of some of these guys, so they wouldn't even think of going out with a girl in real life if she wasn't physically very attractive. They are looking for girlfriends who are way out of their league and I find this shallowness very sad.

Also, some guys are keen to keep up contact between dates because they want to feel like it's a real friendship and that they are special. They almost treat the websites like dating sites! If they phone, text and email escorts between dates, they think it makes them different from all the other guys the girl sees. I simply don't have the time to do this, so I don't, and this is another reason I don't appeal to some guys. My life is not all about my job: my personal life and my friends are separate. I'm not saying I'm not friends with the people I see, but it's different. After all, if I constantly keep in touch with my regulars, whatever would we talk about when we meet?

I know girls who are constantly pestered by their regulars and who also encourage it. I just don't have the time to endure this – there isn't one person in my life at the moment that I would want to speak to every day! I don't mind exchanging a few emails between dates, but I learnt the hard way that too much contact is confusing for guys. People wouldn't call their accountant or solicitor every day, and it's the same thing – men and women pay for an escort to be their friend and companion for a set amount of time. To have constant contact would be too much like a proper relationship and that's not what I offer. Often guys find it difficult to leave the emotional feelings they get while they are with an escort behind when she leaves. Because we offer such intimacy, it's especially difficult with the GFE.

Some guys are constantly on message boards or in the chat rooms, and I just don't think it's healthy to have escorts as such a big part of their lives. Many of them make such a lot of sacrifices to fund their hobby. They are not all rich men. Some clearly don't spend money on themselves, their home or even on holidays; it's all spent on escorts. I once saw a guy who worked stacking shelves in a supermarket – he had saved up all year and probably not had a holiday, just to have an overnight date with me. I've stayed at people's homes to find their towels are threadbare, yet they've paid me £1,500 to visit them!

There is one guy who sees and reviews the same escort every week. It's the most bizarre relationship ever. He is married, too, so I don't know how he has so much time. I think that he's a control freak and he knows that the more he sees her and reviews her, then the more people will understand that she's 'his girl'. Some guys have said they have been put off meeting her because it would be like seeing his girlfriend, and I think that's what he wants. She's about 18, and he's in his sixties, which I find a little disturbing. His reviews of her are just about the conversations they have together, and about him getting her cups of coffee and other mundane daily tasks; it's very odd.

Other guys can't get hold of her to book her. She doesn't mind because she gets all her business from him, so she doesn't need the extra work. He then loves to act almost like her pimp when people enquire about her on the message boards – when they can't get a response from her, he says he will get her to call or email them; it makes him feel important. He sees other girls, but he's totally obsessed with escorts and with this one in particular. It's very sad and I pity him, because he's living in a fantasy world. He has a very big mouth on the message boards, and in the chat room, but I've met him at various work parties (by the way, before you let your imagination run wild, these are not orgies, they're just normal parties and we're probably more behaved than many people at regular office parties!), and he's really shy and hardly speaks to anyone.

Some guys are totally delusional and think they are someone important if they see lots of escorts and write many reviews. It's almost like it's a status symbol and something to be proud of. Who can write the most reviews? Who's seen the most escorts? Some guys are even sad enough to look up to these people. The escorting world can be very bizarre and surreal.

The thing about offering the GFE, where you're seeing people for longer dates and building up a relationship (of sorts) over time, is that guys do become confused and emotions can get involved. I empathise with guys when this happens, because I know they can't control their feelings. For a GFE it's about getting the balance right. You don't want to be cold and clinical, but if you're too affectionate then the guys think there's something more to the relationship. It's incredibly difficult to get the balance right because there's no set rule: everyone is different.

Guys can write reviews on both of the websites I use, and as an escort I have no control over this. The good thing about Northern Angels' reviews is they aren't explicit; they concentrate on the lady as a person. But the negative side of this is that nothing bad can be written, so other members can't warn each other about poor-quality service and any other bad experiences. When someone has a bad date, we can all get tarred with the same brush.

When people whinge about a girl's poor service, I say the same thing, time and time again: they need to do their research, by checking non-biased review sites like Punternet, Punterlink and Captain 69. None of these reviews are to be taken literally, but you can read between the lines and look for similarities in what different people are saying about the same girl. Bad comments aren't to be taken at face value either – it depends whether they are written as constructive criticism or are just plain rude and insulting. And of course, we all have off-days and you can't 'click' with everyone. Generally, reviews by guys who have reviewed several other ladies carry more weight. Often I find that the reviews and the way they're written say more about the guy's personalities who write them than the escort herself.

Like any trade, there are good and bad escorts. There are some who don't care and others who are unreliable, who simply won't return your call or email, or even turn up for a date. Then there are those who take pride in their business – people like me. I've worked hard to build up a good reputation and I always make sure that I'm punctual, well groomed and at my best. In seven years I can count the number of cancellations I've made on two hands. And every time I've had to cancel, I've always compensated the gentleman by giving him extra time or some money off his next date. Interestingly, when it's the other way round and the guy cancels a date with me, it's extremely rare that I'm compensated even though I'm the one out of pocket. I've been compensated maybe four times in my career.

Diary: August 2008

I hazarded a look at my watch because I knew our time was up. He was sweating, penetrating me on top, and he wanted to slow down because he was about to come. 'Go on,' I urged. 'Later,' came the reply. 'Later? What do you mean? I'm leaving in a minute!' I light-heartedly said, looking at my watch. Joking back, he looked at his imaginary watch as if to imply I shouldn't have been checking the time.

I hate the word 'later' – especially when it's referring to me or my date having an orgasm; it's usually said when there's about five minutes, if that, left of my booking or at one in the morning on an overnight date. 'Later' is never convenient. What time can be classed as a minimum time for 'later' and what's the maximum? To me, 'later' suggests hours. It's when the alarm bells start ringing and I know I'm going to overrun.

I don't consider myself a clock-watcher, but my rule is I don't want to be having sex when it's time to go. If my guy has come, I'll happily stay ten or fifteen minutes over time and chat, but after that I go. I don't like people taking the piss, and clients who are still having sex with me five minutes before their time is up are usually serial piss-takers.

Today I met a Northern Angels member, Andy, for a three-hour lunch date. I had my old special on again – buy two hours, get one free (as long as you're feeding me!). I saw him once two years ago for a lunch date and he contacted me recently, asking about a date and looking for any special offers. Cheeky bugger! He's a car salesman... say no more.

So, I gave him my three-for-two, and we arranged a three-hour lunch date at a local hotel. I knew I would recognise him when I saw him, but I still couldn't picture him. He wanted us to meet in the car park, but I suggested he waited in the bar to save either of us loitering around.

I arrived bang on time and strolled confidently into the hotel. Heading towards the bar, I ducked my head and grinned as I saw someone I recognised. I was pretty sure it was him but suddenly I worried about approaching him, in case it wasn't. As I walked into the bar he turned around; it was him, after all... Phew!

I wasn't sure if he was an eager beaver; I couldn't remember. He seemed very relaxed and wasn't in a rush to get to the table, so I ordered a glass of champagne and we sat in the bar and chatted.

Now this guy is the opposite of my guys with SMS – but it's equally bad. Straightaway, he asked me lots of personal questions about how my business was doing and was eager to start talking about me, but not in a polite way. It was quite intrusive, even to the point where he asked me about a client I had seen who was a member on one of the message boards. Obviously, I gave nothing away.

He seemed very relaxed and it was refreshing, but I reminded myself that so many guys who start out like this switch to being eager beavers in the bedroom. We spent around 40 minutes chatting with our aperitifs and I did wonder whether he was actually a news reporter, with all of his intrusive questioning. For once, I really tried hard to steer the conversation away from me and towards him.

Eventually we sat in the restaurant and we were the only ones there. He only ordered a steak, but I asked for a starter too, and then he asked me about my personal life. As if he hadn't already got personal enough! Stupidly, I found myself opening up to him, gassing away about my string of failed relationships – maybe because it was refreshing to find someone interested in me for once!

When I'd finished my food, I was aware two hours had gone by, so even though I fancied a dessert, I declined. If I have a big meal at lunchtime, I make the most of it because usually I don't have anything else when I get home.

He then ordered coffee, which was fine, but straightaway my radar popped up – I knew then he'd try to take the piss and get me to stay longer. I ordered a mint tea and finished it quickly. By the time we'd got to the room and both freshened up, we had 45 minutes left. When he came out of the bathroom, I had made sure I was down to my lingerie so we wouldn't have to take our time undressing.

He poured us champagne, after asking if I wanted it now or 'later'. I had 45 minutes left, so when exactly would 'later' be? I suspect he meant later as in 'later when we've spent hours in bed and both lost track of time...'

Eagerly, he leant in for a slobbery kiss. It was disgusting. Why on earth do guys do this? Quickly, he evened things out by removing his clothes, leaving only his black briefs. Before long we were both naked, him taking the lead as he sucked my breasts and slobbered down my chest (which was quite nice, actually) until he found my pussy. His oral sex felt amazing: now I don't mind slobber down there, just not on my mouth! But he tried to delve his fingers in, and I'm not a fan of that. It's the kind of thing teenage lads do, and once you get a bit older it loses its appeal. It's a bit uncomfortable and it makes me want to pee. I kind of like guys probing at the opening, an inch or so in, but when they try to poke their fingers right up, its not pleasant.

Eventually I had to physically remove his finger and thankfully he took that as a sign that it was my turn and he came back up to kiss me. As he hovered over me, I took the tip of his penis and rubbed it on my clit; he shook, sweated and went bright red as he tried to contain himself.

Gently, I moved him off and onto his back so I could take him in my mouth. 'Careful,' he warned. I wanted him to just come, not because I didn't want to entertain him, but he had been the one wanting to spend longer over dinner. I just don't enjoy a guy coming, then me rushing off; I like to relax afterwards and I'd rather sacrifice a little chatting time to be able to do that. Of course guys often want me to stay over time, and I know I could, but I never do if someone is trying to take the piss.

With five minutes to spare, I got a condom and by the time I'd put it on the clock was ticking like Countdown. He was trying to take his time and tease me. Am I going to have to fake an orgasm to prompt him to come? I wondered. So I groaned louder and panted, then he asked if I'd come.

And that's when he decided he'd come 'later'. After I repeated that I would be off in a minute, I asked what we could do to make him come, so the condom came off and I sucked with vigour. Sixty seconds left. Finally he came, and I moved away and squashed his member between my breasts just as he gushed over them. He then said that I could stay with him that evening in the hotel room. How kind! Er, no...

He wanted us to leave together, and again tried to keep me that little bit longer. Yes, he'd managed it. In true 'take-the-piss-and-get-that-little-bit-more' style he'd managed to squeeze another half-hour out of me. I had better make sure I'm more on the ball next time. I took the rest of the bottle of Moët, which he put in a carrier bag. I looked like a real pisshead. 'How are you going to carry it?' he asked. 'I'll be swigging it from the bottle as we leave,' I replied.

CHAPTER 10:

Captain 69

C aptain 69 is primarily a review site. It's UK-based, but
covers escorts worldwide and has members in many
other countries. Guys can use the site to review a lady's
performance as an escort, and these reviews inevitably help
and hinder our careers. The site consists of male and female
members. Most females are escorts (active and retired) and
most of the men are punters. Male members can review any
working girl or agency worldwide. There's a forum for
discussion, a chat room and various other advertising tools
there. No escort, member or not, can prevent reviews from
being published, and she can't view her own reviews unless
she's a member herself.

I pay for a membership. Fortunately I've over 35 positive
reviews. I'm very selective about the people I see, and I
think this helps me avoid negative reviews. I tell people
straightaway if I don't think I'm the right escort for them; I
won't take on just any job for the money, even if I'm
desperately short of work.

People rate your looks and performance, and then write about their experience. Some ladies get reviews that are very explicit and I always think they say more about the guy and his view of his own sexual prowess than about the escort. It's amazing how different the client's view of the date can be! The guy might say he made her come three times with the noisiest, most satisfying orgasms, thanks to his stamina in the bedroom, but the escort's recollection may be that she didn't come and he suffered premature ejaculation.

Even though I have no control over what's written about me, fortunately my reviews aren't generally of the explicit type. As I offer the 'girlfriend experience', I prefer people to talk about their experience with me as a whole, including my companionship. The common theme of any bedroom action in my reviews is, 'I won't go into detail'. I don't want to be booked or not booked because of my performance in bed; I want people to make their choice based on my personality. Thankfully, most of the guys I see respect my wishes to keep our private time private.

I'll show you how different some of these reviews can be. Here's an example of one of the explicit reviews, and a non-explicit one of mine:

'I wanted a Porn Star Experience with lots of dirty talk, and that's what I got. C seemed to enjoy herself as much as I did. After our first round, it took her a matter of minutes to get me hard again. What followed was an amazing blow job with lots of eye contact. I came in her mouth as she looked at me, smiled and swallowed the lot!'

'It was an extremely high-class experience from one of England's top courtesans, Bea. From the website, telephone calls and emails to her arriving exactly on time – everything was highly professional. When you meet Bea, it's clear from the start that she genuinely enjoys meeting

people and providing them with a very special time. Some
ladies have that easy-going nature and natural charm that
makes them even more attractive in person. The rest of
the evening turned out very nicely too, but you'll get no
details from me. If you want the Bea experience I strongly
recommend that you book well in advance and plan a
minimum of five hours or an overnight.'

The guys on Captain 69 are a different breed. Of course there
are some horrible people on there, too – escorts and guys
alike – but also some real gems. Threads on the Captain
69 forums are often more serious and sometimes quite crude,
such as 'Who offers the best rimming in London?', 'PSE
[Porn Star Experience] recommendations', 'Working girls
offering bareback sex [sex without a condom]' 'Boob jobs:
what guys really think about them', 'Who's got the biggest
tits? Biggest clit?' and so on. But the threads also cover
sport, politics and general world news; sometimes even
amusing jokes.

Captain 69 also has a section called Members' Requests,
where guys can request girls for certain trips and services. I
reply to them if I'm interested. Here's an example of one that
piqued my curiosity – it's one of the dates I've written about.
The ad on the board was from a guy whose pseudonym was
Andy, and it read:

'*Hi!*
Do you fancy enjoying a 24-hour visit to Venice?
I am looking for a slim and busty girl who provides
a good GFE service (DFK and OWO above all) for a
reasonable rate.
Send me an e-mail and let's see...
London based or anywhere else based, doesn't really
matter.'

I love Venice, and I've been fortunate enough to visit twice already with work, so I know my way around a bit. Also, I can fly there from East Midlands very conveniently, so I checked and there were flights available for the dates he requested. DFK means Deep French Kissing, and OWO is Oral Without. I offer both these services, so I thought he was worth replying to. So, I sent him an email – my standard email introducing myself and pointing him to my site; I also mentioned that I offer a GFE, and listed a couple of other qualities that I have. I said that I'm friendly and reliable, and I always finish by saying a response would be appreciated. Many don't even bother to reply, but it's worth replying to some of these requests because sometimes it gets me a job.

Andy replied, and was very keen for me to fly out to Venice. It was a positive sign that he replied so promptly. He wanted to know what he needed to do, and said his budget was £1,000 and that he wanted to meet from 5.30p.m. until late the next morning. That's fine with me. My flight got in at lunchtime, but I could have a few hours to myself to enjoy a shop. His English was so good in his email that I actually thought he was English and wanted me to travel out to Italy with him. I told him I book my own flights and that the total inclusive cost would be £1,300, to cover my flights and transport.

He wanted me to stay at a flat he owns in Italy. He's Italian, and it transpired his real name was Roberto, but doesn't live in Venice. He shares the flat with his brother. He said he was mid-thirties and that I would find him attractive. 'I'll be the judge of that', I thought. Normally, I wouldn't visit someone I've never met before at a private residence, but so long as I can verify the address and the landline number there, then it's usually OK. I told him I would need to speak with him before I could confirm anything. He agreed to give me a call and let me have the personal information I needed.

I always wonder what percentage of time guys will want to spend in the bedroom. Although I enjoy sex on an extended overnight date, I'm not a nymphomaniac, so I wouldn't expect to have sex more than three times – once after we've had a drink and got to know each other, once after dinner and once in the morning. I can hardly ask clients how many times they expect to have sex, so I usually email them in advance to ask what plans they have for our time together. If they really are some sex-crazed addict, they'll mention the sex and maybe say something like, 'Well, I don't imagine we'll get out much', and then the alarm bells would ring and I wouldn't agree to go.

Roberto pleasantly replied suggesting we have a drink and a 'get-to-know' session at his place (this I take to mean sex) and then a leisurely time getting ready for dinner. He suggested a traditional restaurant, and then a wander around the city in the evening before retiring. It sounded perfect to me.

Diary: April 2006

God, I had an absolute nightmare yesterday! I decided that I would check in online for my flight to Venice, giving me a bit more of a lie-in. My flight was at 8.50a.m., and checking in online meant I only needed to be at the gate 30 minutes before. I booked a taxi for 7.45, thinking the traffic wouldn't be so bad then. How the hell would I know? I never drive that time in the morning. That's one of the benefits of being an escort – I don't have to spend hours stuck in rush-hour traffic. Why I didn't ask my taxi driver what time to set off, I have no idea.

Tuesday night, I had my early night planned; I had packed and watched a bit of telly, so I felt suitably relaxed. I decided I would have a shower and wash my hair at about 9p.m., and go straight to bed. However, my plan was foiled when I found I had no water. I willed myself to keep calm despite this obvious crisis: I knew it wouldn't be back on by the morning – last time we had a leak, there was no water for 14 hours. Fortunately, I had a good supply of water left from the last time, so I would have to bath and wash in mineral water. How terribly posh! I'm sure some famous people only bath in Evian. So I put the kettle on to boil. I kissed goodbye to my early night, which would now be replaced by boiling the kettle and spending the evening trying to clean, shave my bits and the mammoth job of washing my hair while hanging my head over the bath with a washing-up bowl and jug.

Suddenly there was a spurt of water from my shower, so I dived in and frantically started wetting my hair and trying to put shampoo on it. As the water spluttered to a final stop, I cursed and begged it to come on just a little bit more. It didn't. Fortunately, the kettle had boiled so I finished washing my hair and shaved in a washing-up bowl that I'd placed in the bath. By the time I dried my hair and got myself ready for bed, it was about 11p.m... Then there was a knock at the door, which I really didn't want to answer because I thought it would be my neighbour wanting to moan about the water. I opened it to find the plumbers standing there, saying the water would be back on at about midday. Of course this was absolutely no use to me! Stressed, I went to bed and set my alarm for seven.

I had a bit of a restless night, but got up without any problems. By the time I had washed in the tub again, it was time for the taxi. My driver was concerned to find that my flight was at 8.50, but he promised he would do his best. That was when I started to worry, but in the back of my mind I kept telling myself it would be fine. I couldn't relax – the traffic was everywhere. It was looking increasingly unlikely that we would make it, so I started making calls to see what other flights were available, but I couldn't find one that would get me there in time. So much for my leisurely afternoon in Venice! I asked the taxi driver if he would wait and see whether I caught my plane. Fortunately, he said he was able to take me somewhere else, if need be.

I flew through to departures with five minutes to spare, where I was stopped and my luggage hauled off to be inspected – apparently I had too many liquid toiletries. I only had my essentials! There was my eczema cream, Gucci perfume and body lotion, Chanel perfume, shower gel, three travel-sized body lotions, hand cream, my face essentials, vaginal lubrication and massage oil, foundation, lip plump, concealer and tinted moisturiser.

The lady took her time in opening my bags. I tried to keep myself under control and said my flight was leaving. They halved the contents of my toiletries. I ran to the gate and arrived out of breath to be greeted by a bunch of airport staff, who casually informed me the doors were closed and the plane had started its taxi to the runway. Teary-eyed, I made my way back through Security, where the kind lady who had taken her time to search my bag looked at me with pity and said, while handing me the toiletries she had confiscated, 'Can you go another day?' 'Er, no', I replied.

I quickly walked through to the ticket desk and stopped to ask BMI about flight times; they informed me they didn't fly there. The only other EasyJet flight was too late. Ryanair had a flight at 3p.m. from East Midlands, but a 12.05 from Stansted. I quickly called and asked my taxi driver if he could get me to Stansted for 11, and he said he could, but the lady at the desk refused to sell me a ticket because she didn't think I'd catch the plane.

I sprinted out to my taxi anyway, and we set off. Like Anneka Rice on some big mission, I just had to catch this flight otherwise I'd have to get a lift back up to East Midlands for the 3p.m. flight and then I would be late, something I absolutely hate. I was praying my client didn't call because I didn't want to worry him unnecessarily.

As time was ticking on, I worried the whole way down but when I called Ryanair they told me the flight was at 12.45, not 12.05 as I had been told at the airport, so I did have plenty of time when I arrived. I just prayed there was still availability and not too much of a queue at the sales desk; I just wanted to be able to relax. I felt knackered as I'd been up since seven, and then stressing and travelling ever since. I felt dirty because I hadn't been able to have a proper shower; I just didn't feel my best. I only hoped I could relax when I arrived and be good company.

I got the ticket, and chastised myself for being so laid-back about getting to the airport in the first place. I had just lost £320 of my earnings – the flight was £220, and the taxi £100. As you can see, I'm more like Bridget Jones than Belle de Jour!

I managed to get a card to give to Roberto (my date) and a magazine before running to the gate to board my flight. Hot and flustered, I must have looked like a madwoman. I had walked so much, and I was tired and frustrated, yet I couldn't sleep at all on the plane because I was still winding down from all the stress. Once we'd taken off, I went straight to the ladies' to apply some make-up to try and make myself look a little bit glamorous. It certainly wasn't how I felt!

Finally, I arrived in central Venice ten minutes before I was due to meet him – I'd been travelling for over eight hours. I nipped into a chemist, looked at their small selection of fragrances and picked one as a present for my date. I always like to take a gift when I'm travelling abroad to see someone, or if I'm seeing someone for a few days. I called Roberto and he said that he would wait outside the bar where we had agreed to meet. I suggested he went inside and ordered a drink for us both.

Then I switched into work mode, put a big smile on my face and put my stress behind me. It's not about pretending to be someone else – I'm still me, but a focused me. Like a director of a company who has to do a presentation – no matter how stressful their day has been, or whatever personal problems they have, they put it all aside and do their job. I go over my little mantra in my head: 'I am confident, happy, sexy, stress-free Bea!' It's about changing my frame of mind. As soon as I walk into the bar, my date is my focus and it's all about how he feels, and how I make him feel: it's not about me.

He was average looking, very tall and skinny, with dark hair, and he was around my age. He hadn't ordered drinks. I told him about my nightmare of a day, and we talked about Venice and his family. He seemed a really nice guy and very politely complimented me on my looks. Well, I think it was a compliment. He said, 'Wow!' It could have been, 'Wow, you look rough!', or 'Wow, you whiff a bit!' or even, 'Wow, you don't look as good as your photos'!

We waited about half an hour before we got a drink. I must have looked like an alcoholic – all I could think was how desperately I needed a glass of wine! He asked if I was hungry, and as he hadn't booked a table until 9p.m., and I hadn't managed to eat much, I decided to have something. So, we ordered a platter to share. He delicately picked at bits of bread and meat, while I tried to make full-on sandwiches with Parma ham and cheese. The ham kept sticking in my teeth – so much for trying to be sophisticated! I was starting to relax and was confident we would have a nice evening. He didn't rush me at all, and we stayed until about 7p.m. before making the move to his flat. It was quite old, full of antique furniture and mismatched random things. He then informed me that his brother was also staying – I wondered what he had told him about me.

I wanted to have a shower, but when I saw the Jacuzzi it seemed like a much better option, as it would help me to relax. In his room I gave him his present, and he was thrilled. We sat on his bed and he leaned in to kiss me. I wanted to be clean before I did anything, so I wasn't very responsive, but suggested we share a bath. It must have taken over half an hour to fill up; disappointingly, it wasn't hot. I stripped off and he just kept saying 'Wow!' so I think it was all good. He stripped off too, and we both got in. I ran my hands over his back, and we caressed each other and kissed, then I started wanking him in the water. After a brief few minutes he came and then hosed me down with the shower. So that was a quick session!

I wore my new giraffe-print dress, with a black cardigan and tan shoes. I was pleased to see that he made the effort and wore a suit. I didn't know what to expect for dinner, but he said his friend had recommended this place and that it was high up and had views over Venice. When we arrived at the 5-star hotel I was impressed – it seemed this would be a bit special. The room was candlelit, with soft music playing. It was very romantic. One side of the restaurant was all glass, looking out over Venice.

We spent the next three hours eating and chatting. He said he had never seen any English girls before, and that he was pleasantly surprised that I wasn't like the Eastern European party girls he saw, who wanted to be out drinking and clubbing all night. After the day I'd just had, there wasn't much chance of that – I'd surprised myself by still being up!

The food was delicious. We had strawberry champagne cocktails with various canapés. I asked him if he liked English food, and he said he didn't think there was any. All I could come up with was cottage pie! When I saw crumble on the dessert menu, I suggested he tried it. Thankfully, he really enjoyed it and, satisfied, we both left at midnight. Back at his flat I met his brother and I was impressed with his good looks (a threesome would be nice, I thought). He was shorter, with glasses; a bit geeky, but in a kind of sexy way, and he wasn't skinny, just in proportion. Roberto joked that his brother would have to inspect me. Yes, please! He was only 22, and was finishing his medical degree.

After a few minutes we left his brother to his studying. Roberto then got me a glass of water, but I suddenly became paranoid he might have put something in it, so I paused and just looked at it. He knew what I was thinking because he said, 'It's not poisonous, you know' and took a swig. I just had to check.

In his room we stripped off, dimmed the lights and I went down on him. Then we swapped around. It felt gorgeous, but unfortunately he didn't do it for long. He got one of his own condoms and slipped it on. I climbed on top of him and ground away for a short while, looking at him in my best sexy way. We then changed to missionary and I wrapped my legs around him really tightly, while nudging his hips down with my feet, holding him tightly while kissing and nibbling his neck. This seemed to do the trick and he came pretty quickly.

I asked him if he could play with my boobs while I used my toy because I was turned on and a bit tipsy! He was thrilled at the idea and I came in about a minute. He made a point of saying how much he enjoyed watching me play with myself – and he was still hard after we finished, so I went down on him again. He enjoyed it for a few minutes and then said he needed to take five minutes' rest. That brought me back to reality, and I suggested we wait until the morning. Thankfully, he agreed, as it was now past 1a.m.

I had to leave at 10.45a.m., so when he offered to set the alarm for 9.30 the following morning, I thought 'perfect'! I kissed him goodnight, thanked him for a lovely evening and hoped I would get a good night's sleep. But I needn't have worried as he didn't snore and kept to his side of the bed. It seemed really late when the alarm finally went off, but it was 9.30a.m. I figured we had about 30 minutes to play.

In the morning it's generally a quicker session, so I just started giving him a blow job. He enjoyed this for a while before saying in his sexy voice, while gently pulling me away, 'I waaaaant a beeeeet of pussy.' Phwoar! I passed him a condom to put on. He lay behind me and groped my breasts while sliding inside me. He had his hands free, one of which was very gently rubbing my pussy. Then he wanted doggy-style, which I like because he could go nice and deep. I glanced up at him through the mirror over his bed, and he was looking at me and getting off on watching us. Eventually he took the condom off, I poured lubricant in between my breasts and he quickly climaxed in between them.

Unfortunately there really wasn't time to hug and relax, so I asked him for a cuppa and dived into the shower. Once I was ready, I barely had time to drink my tea, which had gone cold, before setting off for the airport.

CHAPTER 11:

Crossing the Road Can Be Dangerous

I know many of you will assume my job is dangerous, and it can be, just like crossing the road. But how you choose to do things determines whether a situation is dangerous or not. I'm not saying my safety is 100% guaranteed, but then what is? All I can do is minimise the risks involved. However, I cringe when I think of the dangerous situations I put myself in during younger, pre-escorting days.

What angers me is society's view on my profession, when there are so many women who frequently put themselves in more dangerous and degrading positions socially. Why is escorting so taboo, when you think of the increase in binge-drinking and the state some women get themselves into before going off and sleeping with strangers?

Girls get drunk and wander off from their friends without saying where they're going, and then they go to some random guy's house to have sex with him. That's what I consider dangerous – yet people think my job is far worse. I'm proud to say that I never get myself into an embarrassing state when I'm out socially. In fact, when I'm with my friends, I'm often the one who takes on the role of looking out for everyone, making sure they're OK. Don't get me wrong, I enjoy going out and I love to have a dance, but I'm always aware of what's going on around me and I never go out on the pull. I can't stand the way men think it's OK to grope women and I hate the fact that they often take advantage and look for pissed-up women who might be too drunk to protest. One-night stands don't interest me at all. I've been there and done that, and I don't want any more meaningless sex in my life: I have enough of that with my work.

I'll tell you what I think is dangerous: the number of friends I have who meet guys on the Internet or in the street, and who go to these guys' homes without telling anyone where they are. I'm extremely protective of my friends and some I really worry about. One friend often gets drunk, and then takes a man back to hers and has sex with him. She does this at least once a week, so she probably sleeps with more men than I do! I can go for over a month, sometimes two, without work.

Another friend met someone on the Internet and went to his house to meet him in person for the first time. She was going to stay overnight with him, and of course he said he was sleeping on the sofa. Yeah, right! I asked why she didn't get him to meet her somewhere neutral and she said she would, but she didn't. Needless to say, she had lots to drink and they slept together. I think this is a million times more dangerous than what I do and yet I'm the one that gets judged. How many more will be judging me just from reading this book?

Many women use sex to get what they want at some point in their life, whether it's sleeping with their boss to get ahead, or withholding sex from their husbands because they're annoyed at them. Then there are girls who make a bee-line for DJs and club owners to get various perks, or women who marry for money. They're all being deceitful. At least I'm not trying to be sneaky – people know where they stand with me.

For my safety, I always ensure someone knows where I am when I'm working and who I am with, and I make sure the guy knows that someone knows where I am. I think that's basic common sense. I cannot believe how many escorts don't tell anyone where they're going – there's absolutely no excuse. You need to have common sense and listen to your instincts in this job. If something doesn't feel right, then it isn't.

For three years now, I've also trained in the Japanese martial art of Aikido. I do this to keep fit and to build up my confidence, but also for personal protection. I've recently got my 2nd Kyu (I'm two belts away from black) and go two or three times a week to train. We also learn a lot of self-defence techniques, for knife and gun attacks as well as physical attacks.

A young friend of mine started escorting at 18, and I was extremely concerned when she said that her mum had encouraged her. I think the legal age for escorting should be higher than 18 – in my opinion, at least 21, but preferably 25. At 18 you think you're really grown-up, but you're not. I couldn't discourage her, so all I could do was to advise her on how to be safe. The first piece of advice I gave her was to always tell her mum where she was going, who she'd be with and when to expect her back. And the second most important thing was never to do anything she didn't want to do. Unfortunately, she didn't take my advice on either of these things.

One morning I got a phone call from her mum, who was in tears saying she hadn't come home. I asked her where she had gone and what information she had; all she knew was that she was in Liverpool somewhere. She was supposed to have been back the night before, and by 11a.m. the next day there was no sign of her and her phone was off. I was worried sick, as was her mum. Finally, she called about half an hour later, when she had returned home. She said that the guy had decided he wanted her to stay overnight, and she'd done so without calling her mum, probably because she thought it would be unprofessional to make a call. I had a go at her, but her carelessness and immaturity put a strain on our friendship as I was constantly worried about her.

As an escort it's extremely unprofessional to have your phone on while with a client, but when I've been in a similar situation, I've said that I would be able to stay over but that I need to call my mum/boyfriend/friend to let them know I'm OK and won't be back that evening.

Mostly, I visit hotels, and hotels have to swipe a credit card on arrival, so they know the identity of the person in the room. Nowadays, if you want to pay for a room in cash, hotels are very cautious. I once had a dinner date in Sheffield, and the guy called to tell me he was going to be late because the hotel wouldn't let him check in and pay cash without seeing his passport, so he had to go home, which fortunately wasn't far away, and then come back with his ID. So, at least there's some security there. If I'm going to someone's home, I ask for a landline number and I use this to check that the person is who they say and that they really do live there. If the number is ex-directory, I'll ask for a reference from another girl he's seen and call her to see if he's OK. If none of the above can be done, I usually ask him to book a hotel.

I take a full name, contact number and a booking reference for the hotel. The more hoops you make people jump through, the more it puts off anyone dodgy. There are plenty of girls who won't even take a name or number. I don't do anything with the booking reference, it's just one of the hoops, but sometimes I call and ask to be put through to the gentleman. Then, if he has given a false name, I'll find out.

When people give a false name, it's not necessarily because they are dodgy; it's usually because they're paranoid. Recently, I had a dinner date booked near Birmingham. When I spoke to the guy, I asked his name and he said that the hotel was 'booked under' James Smith. This told me he hadn't used his real name, so I asked what his real name was, and he said James Smith. He made me feel a bit silly for asking, like it was obvious.

I didn't believe him, but I knew I could check it with the hotel. I decided to put my name check into action by calling and asking to be put through to Mr Smith. When he answered, I said, 'It's meeeeeeee!' 'Who's me?' came the reply, and I realised I had the wrong person. 'Ooops, sorry,' I said and hung up. Then I called my client on his mobile and said I had been put through to Mr Smith and that it wasn't him. I asked what his real name was, and he told me, but I said he'd have to wait while I sent that information through to my friend, who always knows where I am. He apologised and said he hadn't considered that side of things.

I'm always learning from my mistakes and tightening up safety procedures. I used to give out my real first name and I made the mistake of letting a regular have my surname to book some flights to New York. We would be staying for five nights and he had paid me a deposit. I'd been seeing him for about two years, so you'd think after that amount of time that I could trust him, but what happened next proved that I couldn't rely on my instincts 100%, no matter how well I thought I knew someone.

He was an Asian guy in his thirties, quite good looking and not demanding at all. I used to look forward to seeing him because we got on very well. It started off as an overnight once a month and then progressed to a two- or three-night stay once a month. We would meet, have dinner and sometimes watch a movie. When we went away for a few days, he would buy me gifts and beauty treatments.

Many guys don't like any kind of other entertainment on a normal overnight date – they want you to be 100% focused on them. This can be emotionally draining, so I thought it was great that he would suggest a movie. He was very chilled. When we had fun in bed, although he wasn't interested in pleasuring me, it didn't matter because it didn't take me long to please him.

I was very excited about our New York trip, and he was happy to pay a deposit so I could block that week out of my diary. Then he cancelled the day before we were due to fly. Unfortunately he lost the deposit, as it was such short notice and I'd had other enquiries for that week, which I'd turned down.

Then a good friend I know through escorting told me about an Asian man who had stalked her friend (who's a bit ditsy) and it transpired this was the same guy. I had to think long and hard about whether I wanted to keep on seeing him. You may think that this was a silly thing to do, but he was a good client: he'd never pestered me and he was bringing me a good chunk of income on a monthly basis. I was glad to be made aware of the other lady's problems, but she had made a big mistake. She made arrangements to see him as a 'friend', even though she had not met him as a client, which is something I wouldn't do.

She was in London and told him where she was staying, but then she changed her mind and said she no longer wanted to meet him. He pestered her with calls, on her mobile and at the hotel. Obviously, this was very inconvenient. He then said he would be waiting outside for her and although she asked the hotel to stop directing the calls through, he persistently called her mobile and threatened her. He said he could find out where she lived, and she was terrified.

I decided if he tried to do anything like that to me, I would just ignore him and he would soon get bored. Generally, I think I'm quite a good judge of character, so I didn't feel threatened. I genuinely thought that although this man clearly had a screw loose somewhere, he was harmless where I was concerned. So, we arranged to meet for a few days in London. I was very blasé as we had met so many times in the past and stupidly, and as I felt guilty that he'd lost his deposit before, I didn't make him pay in advance this time. I wasn't concerned that we hadn't discussed what we would be doing during our stay in London, but as I was packing I called him and left a message asking what clothes to bring. He then started messing around, text messaging me, so I knew he had his phone with him, but he wouldn't pick up when I called. I left him a message saying that I wouldn't set off until I'd spoken to him, so it was in his best interests to call me, but he had decided to play a little game with me and I think it was all because he felt bitter about losing his money from the New York trip.

He then accused *me* of pestering *him*, and text messaged to tell me not to contact him again. I sent one back saying OK, and that was my last contact with him. Over the next few days he repeatedly called me and sent abusive texts. I never answered his calls or returned his messages. He texted me my home address, and told me a date and time when he would be there. I ignored all his efforts and did not fear him. If he turned up at home, I would just call the police. I live in a secure apartment and it's like Fort Knox, so I wasn't worried he would get in. Even if he did, there's no way I would let him into my apartment.

I have kept a birthday card from him, which tickles me every time I read it. He wrote:

You are a super woman. Great looks, super body, humour. Fantastic in bed, what else does a man want?

I have never met a woman who eats so much and looks great.

Long may we be good friends and the rest.

I love and enjoy your company.

Any man just needs to look at you and SPARKS fly around his pants.

For a couple of years he called and texted me at least once a week. A few years ago, he sent me a self-addressed envelope with his mum's address, asking me to refund the deposit he had lost when he cancelled our New York trip. I saved this address in case I ever need to take it to the police. What a plonker he was, giving me his mum's address! The calls and messages became less frequent as he got bored because I wasn't giving him any response.

What I learnt from this experience was never to give out my first or last name, even to my regulars, no matter how much I think I can trust them. I use a pseudonym for my first name and I never give out my surname. I book my own flights. Clients have to transfer money to me, via my business bank account, but I still don't give out my name, just the account details, or I use PayPal, the online money transfer system.

A couple of years ago, I met an American guy at the Dorchester in London for a dinner date. He had booked and paid for a room for me, but he was staying elsewhere. Small and rotund, he looked about 50. I remember something bugged me quite early on. I arrived very early at the hotel and made a call to my friend Nat outside. We talked about lots of personal things, including work, and I noticed a short, fat guy lingering by the entrance, but thought nothing of it. When it was nearly time for me to arrive, I called the client and the guy who was lingering answered his phone. That was extremely freaky, and it set alarm bells ringing – it suggests someone with a controlling nature.

The evening went well, as did the time in the room. The only thing was that he tried to stay longer than the four hours for which he had booked and paid. I mean, I was OK with 20 minutes extra, but after that I wanted to sleep. He got a bit short with me. With him paying for the room, I couldn't just up and leave – that made things a bit awkward. He then requested I visit him in Paris for a couple of days and for two nights in Monte Carlo the week after. I told him I would book the flights and gave him my bank details, minus the name, so that he could pay me a deposit (this was before I had a business bank account). He called me numerous times to say he was unable to make the payment and that he needed my surname. I wouldn't give in, and eventually he said the money had gone through. I was so thrilled when he told me we'd be meeting at the Ritz! I had always wanted to stay at the Ritz and go to Monaco, so I was really excited.

I am always dubious until people pay a deposit because there are so many timewasters and so many guys in a little fantasy world – they enquire, but simply haven't got the money. Some say they're going to take you to exotic places just because they think you'll treat them differently, and they'll get more out of you on a date because you're hoping to impress them so you can be taken to the places they've tempted you with.

Anyhow, this guy did pay the deposit for both trips, so I booked my flights and he gave me the confirmation for the Ritz and our hotel in Monaco. Both hotels looked amazing. I found them on the Internet and eagerly perused their websites. I remember thinking, 'This is what my job's all about: I'm living the dream!' – although of course it would be nice to be able to frequent these places and pay my own way rather than relying on my clients to take me!

A lot of people don't realise there's so much travel involved in my job and they're often surprised when they ask where I've been for work and I reel off a few of the places: Zurich, Milan, Venice, Rome, Hong Kong, Dubai! I get a real buzz from travelling abroad to see clients and for me, this is what being a high-class escort is all about.

I touched down in Paris and got a taxi to the hotel. It felt great to be able to say 'the Ritz, please'. When we pulled up, it was everything that I'd imagined it to be. All the staff treated me like royalty, opening doors and wanting to help me with my small suitcase; I was mesmerised. My client came down to meet me, and took me up the grand gold staircase. The hotel typified luxury in every way, from the large chandeliers and gold railings and trimmings to the fabulous, huge, exotic flower displays and immaculately-presented staff. The room we had was quite small, but I'm sure it must have been ludicrously expensive. There was a large, French-style window with shutters, and the beds and décor were luxurious and classic. It was a shame we were only staying one night, but I wanted to make the most of it.

We went straight out for a walk around the streets of Paris: we walked to the Louvre and then went on a big wheel with views over the city. Afterwards, we stopped at a little café and sat outside, as it was a beautiful day, before heading back to the hotel, where I showered to get ready for our evening out. The bathroom was spacious and beautiful; all the fittings were gold and there was marble everywhere. There was a double sink and fluffy, luxurious peach robes, embroidered with The Ritz logo. If only my bathroom at home could be like that! I remember thinking 'I'm going to pinch all the freebies here'! My date kindly said I could take all the bottles in the bathroom, along with the shoe shiner, slippers, sewing kit and flannel, all with the printed Ritz logo, as souvenirs. I imagined how nice it would be to be there on my own, or with a friend or a boyfriend.

Our next trip was to Monaco, and just ten days after our return from Paris, I was flying out to Nice. We spent the afternoon on the beach in Cannes, but I was thoroughly embarrassed by this loud American, with a huge swollen belly sticking out of a cropped T-shirt. He looked pregnant! Men should never be allowed to wear cropped T-shirts, especially if they are overweight. It was a relaxing afternoon, and we ate lunch in a restaurant overlooking the beach. It was wonderful.

The hotel was gorgeous, high up on the side on the cliff face with views of the town below. It was my first time in the south of France and I couldn't believe I had never been before. There were two outdoor pools with stunning views out to sea. The hotel room was quite basic, but I suspect that because of the location it would have been very expensive. The first night there we ate in the hotel, and ended up having eight courses! I was stuffed. I had worn a glamorous dress as I knew we were going to the casino, and I waltzed in, Sharon Stone style, enjoying the turning of heads. Feeling lucky, I frivolously put lots of chips over various black-and-red boxes at the roulette table. We did quite well, but I'm not sure I'd have been so blasé with my own money!

The next day we drove to St Tropez. We had been told that he wouldn't be able to eat out in the restaurants wearing shorts, so we went on a mission to find some trousers. When he finally found some, he insisted on keeping them on in the shop before he had paid for them, and he spent about ten minutes trying to sit on the security tag remover. It was very comical! On our last day, he had to leave earlier than me, so I spent the morning by the pool admiring the picturesque view, drinking it all in and making the most of the experience before returning to rainy England.

I'd had a wonderful couple of days. Why is it that the nutters are so pleasant to go away with? Before he left, he'd mentioned something cryptic about life being a journey, not a destination, and to enjoy the ride. I thought nothing more of this until I returned home and received a postcard from Cannes: it had my full name and address on it, plus the quote. He didn't sign it, but obviously he didn't need to. He'd sent it while we were away.

He then emailed me and tried to arrange to meet again. I ignored him. He asked if it was because of the postcard, and said there was no way he would have sent money without checking me out. That was fine, but he was obviously another control freak – he didn't need to make a point of telling me he'd looked me up. I never responded, and I wasn't worried – he had more to lose than me. At the end of our date, I left the hotel after him, so I still have a copy of the bill, with all his office addresses and details of his business partners.

A fellow escort once told me always to take my passport with me everywhere, even to the bathroom, and to sleep with it under my pillow. The key thing about safety is to make sure you're always on the ball. That means not getting drunk, so you can keep your wits about you. I'm not saying I never get tipsy, but I try not to, especially with people I haven't seen before.

On one overnight date in London I was given champagne when I arrived, and then we went out and had a taster menu at a Michelin-starred restaurant, with wine to accompany each of the dishes, so I did feel quite tipsy by the time we got back to the room. My client was in a hyperactive mood and asked if I minded if he had a joint. I wouldn't have agreed to him doing any other drug, but I have the odd joint myself so I didn't mind it, and I thought it might help chill him out. I have only ever had a joint with someone twice on a date and would never touch any other drugs, or knowingly see anyone who was on drugs, not even Viagra.

While we were having sex, he put his hands loosely round my neck. I pushed them out of the way, but then he put his hand over my nose and mouth. Then I pushed him away and he apologised, but it was too late. He had made me feel uncomfortable and I abruptly stopped our play-time and said I was going to sleep. I didn't feel scared, because although it sounds scary, my instincts didn't tell me to be fearful. If he'd been forceful then I would have been terrified, but he seemed to just want to see if it was something I was 'into' or not. Had I been near home, I would have probably left. Recently, I got a call from him about a date, and I will see him again. He apologised profusely for his behaviour on our last date and said he wasn't into anything weird. His voicemail said, 'Hi, it's the Boston Strangler'! Although this time I will be making sure he doesn't start smoking his wacky baccy!

In seven years of escorting, the only time I have been

genuinely scared is when a French guy who'd been acting very oddly – which I'd initially put down to nerves – was lying next to me with his arm around me. He'd come to visit me at a hotel, where I was staying in London. I was snuggled into his chest, so couldn't see his face. Although he looked younger, he said he was 50. To make conversation, I asked what he'd done for his 50th birthday. He told me he had gone to the shop, bought a bottle of fizzy water – which he'd pretended was champagne – and a porn magazine, and had gone home to masturbate. Without looking up, I asked why he hadn't had a party with his friends. He said he didn't have any and that he had killed them all, one by one. The last bit was said very slowly and my heart lurched into my stomach. I jumped off the bed and told him to leave. He insisted that he was only joking, but I had a bad feeling and panicked, asking him to leave immediately. I spent the next thirty minutes shaking and sobbing. Why anyone would 'joke' about killing their friends, I have no idea.

Then there's the safe-sex aspect. As soon as I started escorting, I got myself checked out at the clinic and received the all-clear. I told them I was working as an escort and they were very helpful, offering to give me Hepatitis B jabs and giving me good advice. They always gave me a bag of free condoms, which was great considering how expensive they are in the shops. There are things I can catch from kissing and from offering oral sex without a condom, but I have always been clean. And if I'm not sure of someone's hygiene, then I don't go there. Like every escort, I made a choice about my services and I've stuck to it. I can understand why girls don't kiss or offer oral without, but they don't get as much work and in my opinion you can't offer a GFE and not kiss! Girls who don't kiss or do oral sex without a condom mostly get short meetings with clients who just want sex. Some guys don't give me oral sex – I'm sure they think that because of my job I might be dirty!

There are girls who don't use condoms, and in the past I've been offered more money to have sex without one. I refused. Some girls get amazing reviews, with clients rating them a 9 or 10 for looks when their photos tell a different story, and that's usually because they're not using condoms.

When I first started out, I was careless and slept with two guys without condoms. We'd used them initially, but then got lost in the moment and just had sex without. I saw both men regularly and was genuinely very fond of them. When one guy told me he'd caught something from me, I was mortified. I went to the clinic, only to be told I was fine. It transpired his wife had been sleeping with someone at her local gym and he'd caught it off her! It didn't occur to him he might have caught it that way and he obviously assumed, because of my job, that it was from me. Thankfully, that brought me back to reality and I have always used condoms since. Occasionally they have split, but I've never had any problems when I've been checked out.

Most of the guys I see are frequent users of escorts and either only see escorts, or they're married, or have a partner. Generally, they are not people who sleep with multiple partners without protection. I get myself checked out about once every three months and I've always been fine, touch wood!

Diary: February 2008

'Make love to me!' It was an order, not a request — and I was not in the mood. I think it's incredibly rude to order anyone to do anything. Clearly, this guy didn't care if I wanted to have sex or not, and I felt sad that I'd misjudged his character. Only 20 minutes earlier I'd told him that I was sure he wouldn't want me to just go through the motions when I didn't actually want to have sex with him. Obviously, I was wrong.

We'd had an uncomfortable conversation half an hour earlier when he'd asked too many personal questions about my work. I should have steered the conversation towards something safer, but I didn't, and then he asked if I would go away with him for a few days as 'friends'. In other words, after this initial paid trip, he was looking for freebies. He said that I must become friends with my clients, or I wouldn't be able to provide the level of intimacy that I offer. Guys can find it hard to leave their emotions behind after a date has ended, and some call and email me and think we'll meet up for coffee and be 'friends'. I have to explain that I don't become 'friends' with my clients and that I kept things separate. I always hate having to explain this as it sounds like I am a cold person, but I'm not – I just haven't the time to be friends with everyone I see, and the only way I can handle my job is to keep a clear division between my work and personal life. He seemed to think this would be difficult because of the emotions involved in a GFE, but I explained I'd tried it before and let people cross the boundaries and things got confusing for both parties.

Where do you draw the line? Would he expect sex if we went away as 'friends'? Then there's the awkwardness of always having to ask if any future dates are paid bookings. It doesn't work, so I never let anyone get that close. I told him that when I had free time, I went away with friends and family; I could tell he was disappointed I wasn't going to be his 'friend'. I despise the 'F' word now – it's so false, and so many guys I meet don't know the true meaning of the word 'friend'.

He also asked if it was difficult for me to detach from my emotions when I have sex at work. Well, it's quite easy (and it happens subconsciously), especially as sex is expected of me. However, when someone is ordering me to do something and clearly doesn't care how I feel, I can't possibly have any feelings or emotions for that person. If they don't care enough to want me to enjoy myself as much as them, it creates resentment. And he was certainly no gentleman.

This was Adam, a guy I'd previously met for a dinner date in Manchester. He demanded I kiss him before I'd even spoken to him! This was our second date and we were to spend two nights in

Barcelona. On the first morning, he demanded I stroked him and I told him I wasn't in the mood. You can't get more girlfriend-like than that, can you? Two hours later, he demanded that I make love to him. In my mind, you make love with people you love and you have sex with those you don't. It was clear that he had misunderstood my job description. Clients have absolutely no right to demand sex, hugs, kisses, love or anything at all for that matter. I am naturally a very affectionate person, but only when people are respectful and treat me as a lady.

He'd promised a relaxing, fun couple of days. He met me at the airport, but even though I was weighed down with my handbag, duty-free purchases and suitcase, he didn't offer to help carry anything. The hotel was beautiful, though: overlooking the marina on one side and the beach on the other. Looking back, I think he was expecting me to have sex with him when I arrived, which I would never do, even with my regulars. It's not what I offer. I sell my companionship, and anything that happens sexually is by mutual agreement.

It was three in the afternoon and I'd been travelling since 8a.m. I looked over the balcony and he put his arms around me and wanted to kiss me. My heart sank and immediately I was on edge. He was going to be 'one of those' – someone who wants to be constantly touching me in some way. It's very exhausting.

I mentioned I was hungry, as all I'd had was a bag of crisps on the plane. He suggested room service, but after all the travelling I said I'd like to go out and get some fresh air, so we left the hotel and had a wander. He insisted on holding my hand. We settled on an outdoor restaurant – it was exciting to be in Spain with lovely warm sunshine, especially having left a cold and miserable February morning in England. After eating we took a walk around the marina and sat in a café for a drink. He didn't stop talking, and already I knew that I would find him mentally exhausting. I like to be able to have a break in conversation without any awkwardness, a companionable silence. Without this, I can't fully relax.

My head started to throb and the dull headache that had started over lunch progressively worsened. I told him that I needed to lie down for an hour and rest. He seemed fine with that, and went for a walk. I wondered if I was wrong about him – maybe he could be quite chilled after all? He left me for an hour and a half, but I didn't sleep as some builders nearby were making a racket. Nevertheless, it was good to just lie down and have some peace and quiet without the pressure of constant conversation. Once the Nurofen kicked in, I was raring to go!

When he came back, I was in the bathroom. I saw his shadow pass by the glass door and he obviously found the bed and room empty. The light was on in the bathroom and, without knocking, he came to the door and I saw his hand reach for the handle. He was about to come in and he must have known I was in there! I was on the loo and shouted to him that I was in there, so thank goodness he didn't. A guy should respect a girl's privacy. I always lock the door if there is a lock because it's surprising how many times I've been away with guys and they've just wandered in while I've been on the loo, like a married couple. For me it's simple: door open, it's OK to enter. Door closed, it's not. My bathroom time is my bit of privacy.

We both showered and got ready for dinner. Neither of us wanted to wait until 8.30 to eat, but it seemed that nowhere was open any earlier. We had decided to try the hotel restaurant. The food wasn't great – it was one of those places that gave the illusion of being a top-class restaurant, but wasn't. However, Adam's sea bass looked amazing. I wasn't keen on the fishcake I'd chosen, so he kindly gave me a piece of his fish. When the waiter saw I had left my dish, he apologised and asked what I'd like instead. After seeing and tasting the sea bass, I asked for the same as Adam. When mine came with no sauce and some greasy chips on the side, I was frustrated but wasn't about to complain again, so I made do. As food and dining is a big part of my job, it disappoints me when the cuisine is poor.

After polishing off three courses, I was enjoying the rest of my wine when Adam asked if I was done. I'm not 'done' when I still have a half-glass of wine! It was clear that he was impatient to leave, so I quickly finished off the rest of my wine as he disappeared to the loo. Back at the room we had standard, no-nonsense sex. A few minutes of kissing, I went down on him, he went down on me, then sex for a couple of minutes in missionary. We were both tired so it suited us. It was around 12 when we settled to sleep.

The room was stuffy and there was no air conditioning. I told him I liked my own space when I sleep, which I think disappointed him, but aside from the nightmares I have, it's a way of reminding my clients that we are not a 'real' couple. I don't want them getting tempted in the night! But I'm so used to sleeping on my own anyway that I prefer to have my own space and this usually allows me to get a better night's sleep.

However, this time I couldn't sleep and had a restless night because the room was stuffy. In the morning I was exhausted – no way was I up for sex! When he tried, I told him I was tired and not in the mood.

It was then that he demanded I stroke him. Demanding things from me is not acceptable at the best of times, especially not when I'm feeling tired and snappy. I told him 'no', that I was tired, and then I apologised. I decided I'd have a siesta in a few hours to sort myself out, and I'd make it up to him after that. It was obvious that he was in a mood because I hadn't given him what he wanted. Tough! We sat having breakfast and that's when we had the awkward conversation. He seemed in no rush to get out for the day and spent over an hour talking about his 'ex' wife and asking me about my job. He then said he needed to make some private calls, so I left him in the dining room and went back to the room.

It was all very odd, because when he came back he told me about a house he was doing up, in a village 80km from Barcelona, and explained that he needed to get all the piping in place before the plumber arrived. I couldn't understand what had been so private about that call, if that's what he'd been talking about, and I strongly suspected he was lying, but I wasn't sure why. He said he'd have to go and sort it out, and asked if I would be OK. Let me think about that: I have my own suite in a gorgeous hotel, the weather's beautiful and there's a spa, beach and marina on my doorstep! I told him I'd be fine. He said he might be able to come back that day, but would have to leave again at six in the morning. I said fine, but told him not to disturb me at 6a.m. There's no way I'd be in the mood for his demands at that time in the morning.

That was the point at which I was ordered to 'make love' to him. I wondered if he was pretending that he wasn't going to be around later, so I'd have sex with him there and then. I half-expected him to have sex with me and then decide not to go to his house, and that would have left me stuck with him, resenting him for the rest of our stay. I did have sex with him, though, because I had to assume he was telling me the truth when he said he was going. Because men can successfully lie to their wives, I think they assume they will be able to lie to me, but I often see right through them. Sometimes I say something and sometimes I don't – it depends on the situation.

I don't distrust men in general, and I'm not paranoid with the boyfriends I have had (all of them have known about my profession), but I can generally spot a liar, probably thanks to the time I spent with my boyfriend James, who was a compulsive liar, years before.

Anyhow, I digress. My client Adam was paying me for two days and I'd only seen him for one, so at least if I had sex with him I could chill for the rest of the day and evening on my own. But it would still have been kinder for him to ask, rather than demand. He asked me what I wanted him to do for me, but one look at me and he didn't wait for an answer. I just thought, 'get on with it'! And it must have shown on my face. I suggested going for lunch before he left, but he decided he was going to go. So he packed up his things, paid me the remainder of the cash for my trip, and we said our goodbyes and he went off and settled the hotel bill.

Something was extremely odd about it all. I kept expecting him to 'surprise' me and come back, and I wasn't keen on that idea, so I stayed out of the room until 10p.m. I had a wonderfully relaxing day. I sunbathed, went to the spa and treated myself to a facial and massage before going out for dinner at a Chinese restaurant on the marina.

He texted around 10p.m.:

'Bea... are you OK? Hope you have had a battery-charging day away from my demands (sorry) I am still in the thick of it... always been too ambitious X'

I was relieved he wasn't coming back, and texted him to say I was off to bed. I still half-expected him to be in the room when I got there. Again, I didn't sleep well, partly because I was wondering whether he might just turn up at any moment. It crossed my mind that he might have been spying on me – I was a bit paranoid because the situation seemed so strange.

I suspected that he was still with his wife, even though he'd said they were separated, and that maybe she was going to the house, so he had to get back there. Alternatively, perhaps he realised that I wasn't going to be his sex slave and obey his sexual demands. Why else would he pay me so much money and then disappear? Sometimes I find people with money are used to always getting what they want, and I think he was one of those people.

The next morning I went down for a hearty breakfast and took a leisurely stroll along the beach, before heading back to the airport. So I ended up having a relaxing stay, after all!

He never contacted me to make sure I got home safely.

CHAPTER 12:

Boyfriend Number Two – Alex

I joined a scuba group in Nottingham in 2002, to try to make some local friends. Escorting can be very lonely, and although I'd met a couple of other escorts, they weren't really my type of people so I rarely socialised with them.

Two clients had raved to me about scuba diving, and whenever I went into town, I passed a scuba school less than a mile from where I lived, so one day I decided to drop by. The owner asked what I did for a living, and I couldn't think quickly enough to lie, so I told him the truth. He was a friendly guy and didn't mind at all, so I decided there and then to sign up for a course to get the Open Water scuba qualification.

At the time I was still with Kenny, and although I wasn't happy, I wasn't on the lookout for a new boyfriend. I'd gone to the scuba school to meet some local girls to hang out with, and I came to really enjoy the regular meets on a Tuesday night and our social time in the pub afterwards. I then signed up for a week's scuba diving in Egypt, where I would complete my qualification.

When I first met Alex, I didn't really notice him until one night when we got chatting at the pub. I was instantly drawn to him and very physically attracted too, and I couldn't understand why I hadn't noticed how good looking he was before. He was also very funny and friendly. Alex was a couple of years older than me, but not my usual type. He was tall, blond and had an eight-year-old boy from a previous relationship. We clicked and I was really looking forward to my trip to Egypt, as he was going too. He had a girlfriend and I was with Kenny, but I thought a bit of harmless flirting would be OK. I couldn't wait to go away and spend more time with him, and he never asked me what I did for a living.

I hadn't told anyone in my scuba group apart from the owner, Jim, but unbeknown to me he was a huge gossip, and he had spread the word. I just didn't want people to judge me – I wanted them to like me for the person I am. No one ever asked me what I did for a living, and now I know that when people don't ask, it's usually because they already know.

During the holiday Alex and I became very close. He was so charismatic, and I just wanted to be around him all the time. I was sure that the feeling was mutual – we spent hours chatting and it transpired that he too was unhappy in his relationship. He finished with his girlfriend shortly after we came back from Egypt in October, and in December I dumped Kenny. As soon as Kenny realised his free meal ticket was gone, he hounded me and my friends to try and get me to take him back again, but I knew, there and then, that I would never go out with anyone tight again.

One night Alex came back to mine for a coffee after our Tuesday pool session, and we ended up sleeping with each other. He told me that he knew I was an escort (and that everyone at the scuba centre knew), and that he could never go out with one. I was saddened that he'd waited until after we slept together to tell this, because I'd thought this was the start of something special. I'd given myself to someone I had real feelings for, and I was really gutted; I felt cheated and used. I spent the night explaining about my work and hoping to change his mind; I told him the sex I had at work was meaningless and that they got my body, but not my heart. I told him that I didn't even sleep cuddled up with these guys – I'm on the opposite edge of the bed, hanging on for dear life.

The next week I invited him to visit my uncle's farm. My brothers and sister were going down too, my cousins would be there and it was a guaranteed fun party weekend. He accepted my offer and we drove down together. The first night, after a few beers, he told me he could easily fall in love with me. I was thrilled because I saw him as a potential life partner – I'd never had feelings like that for anyone previously or, as a matter of fact, since.

At my suggestion, he moved in with me straightaway. He did need prompting to start paying towards the mortgage and bills, but he was extremely generous, and as soon as I mentioned the mortgage we came to an arrangement. I fell in love with him very quickly and I really thought I had found 'the one'. At times it was difficult to go out to work, because really, I only wanted to be with him and I started to find the sex part of my work very difficult. I would close my eyes and try to pretend I was with him. I'd nip to the loo when I was working and text to say I loved him and was thinking about him. I'd leave him little notes that he'd find when he went to bed, wishing him sweet dreams. When I got back from an overnight date I would literally jump on him, if it was the weekend and he was at home in bed. It was almost like my work was foreplay, and I'd ravish him when I got home.

He used to say he'd try to block out my work, and not think about it, which was fine. Sometimes I'd ask for advice, and sometimes I'd forget I was talking to a boyfriend and perhaps say a little too much, but it never seemed to be an issue. Unfortunately, after about five months we started arguing quite badly. He always tried to persuade me that it was normal for couples to argue, just as Kenny had, so for months I tried to cope with it. My work was never mentioned when we argued, so I don't think it was an issue for him, but I began to fall out of love because the arguing was making me miserable and I told him so.

The only argument we had relating to my work occurred when we were due to go on holiday for a week. I was worried about missing out on bookings, so I wanted to leave my phone on and take calls in the UK until we flew out of Gatwick. He argued it was my holiday time and I should switch off, but I said that if I could confirm just one job for when I got back, it would mean I could relax more on holiday: I had nothing in my diary, and I'm uncomfortable spending money when I'm not earning it. I said that when we got on the plane I would switch my phone off, but we argued so much about it that in the end we really weren't sure whether to go or not. The holiday was an expensive, all-inclusive break, but I don't like being told what to do. I thought he was being ridiculously unreasonable under the circumstances.

As it happened, I did get one call and I discreetly excused myself to take it. Alex glared at me, but there was no way I was going to ignore it. The call lasted no longer than a minute and was a waste of time, but it could have been a genuine booking. When I sat back down, it was clear he had the hump. What a great way to start the holiday! Our time away was strained, and when we got back home the arguing continued.

I don't think he's a bad person, but I was unintentionally bringing out the worst in him and I couldn't understand why. I felt he resented me. I suggested couples counselling, because I was desperate to try to make things work; I didn't want another failed relationship under my belt, I wanted to settle down. He wasn't interested. I suggested we both save to travel for a year, and we decided that would be 'make or break' time. He opened an account for us and we began to save.

One day when he was drunk he admitted that he was jealous

of me, which explained the resentment I felt from him. It seemed like he hated me most of the time. He said he was jealous of my home, my family and my friends. He didn't have a good relationship with his family and they weren't close like mine, but he could have bought a house if he'd wanted to, and he seemed to have lots of friends, although they were more acquaintances that he'd known from school. The first Christmas he spent with me and my family, my mum bought him a stocking and filled it with goodies like she still does for us 'kids'. He said it was the first stocking he'd ever had, that he was overwhelmed, and that he felt more welcome visiting my mum and dad than he did with his own parents.

When it got to the stage that I was staying away from home just to get away from the arguing, I knew I had to end it. He shouted all kinds of abuse at me, so I walked out again, and didn't return for a couple of hours. By the time I got back, he had left and taken his things. If we hadn't argued so much, I would seriously have considered finishing escorting and settling down with him; the more I was falling for him, the more difficult I found my work. To be cuddling on the sofa and then have to get up and get ready to see another man was awful! I really didn't want to go on my dates, but I never cancelled them because I didn't want to let the client down and I had to earn a living.

Of course when the arguments were really bad, work would be a welcome relief as I could focus on someone else, someone who would make me feel appreciated, and I could forget how unhappy I was in my relationship. At times like those, I knew I couldn't stop escorting, because the people I saw on my work 'dates' made me feel happy and good about myself. I know Alex found it very difficult when I was travelling abroad and staying in exotic hotels; he must have wished he could have afforded to take me to places like that, and I wished that too. I don't think he believed I would rather have been with him in all those places – I always called and kept in touch with him whenever I could when I was away, and I missed him like crazy.

Once he moved out, we saw each other a couple of times. When dropping me back at mine one evening, he paused at the door and turned back to me and said, 'I don't suppose you fancy a shag, do you?' Of course I did! Once he moved out, the tension between us eased and we could have possibly worked things out if he'd persevered, but then I asked him for the key back and he assumed I didn't want to see him anymore. That wasn't the case – I just wasn't sure what would happen with the two of us. When I was liaising with him about splitting the money we had saved, I found out he had been ripping me off for about six months, and I never got the full amount I'd saved back. I was really disappointed in him because I trusted him implicitly. I didn't care about the money – what hurt the most was the fact that it was premeditated and the mutual trust and respect that I thought was there wasn't.

When I finished with Alex, I realised this was a turning point in my life. Like a lot of women, I liked being part of a couple, but I found I wasn't worried about being on my own again. My confidence had grown and I felt strong as a person. I was literally buzzing from excitement from being single and having no stress in my life. Once again, my focus was back on my work. My jobs have thrown up some real gems over the years – not only do I get to go on some amazing dates for work, I get paid for it and there's minimal stress!

Diary: March 2008

'Hello stranger, how are you doing? Think it's about time we met up, babes . . .'

This was the text message I received from Simon, a very successful businessman, who works extremely hard. He goes through phases – I'll see him a few times, and then I won't hear anything for ages. We first met when I had just started escorting, and he's one of the few guys that I really fancied, physically and mentally. He'd never seen an escort before and with me being a novice, it meant we were both sussing things out. I actually fancied him so much that I agreed to go out on a non-paid date with him, but this never came to fruition. He also wanted to take me to the Maldives, but he didn't want to pay me anything for the trip and I couldn't afford to take time off as I was in debt, so that was that.

Then I didn't hear from him for about five years. When he

contacted me again, he'd been married and divorced, had a spell in rehab and his mum had just died. His divorce cost him thousands and I told him it would have been cheaper for him to see me during that time than to have got married! He seemed surprised that I'd remembered him. Obviously I don't remember everyone I see, but I often recognise a face or a name if I see them again, and I remembered him because I had fancied him. He had a Porsche and I remember thinking 'why can't I have a boyfriend like him?' I remembered the tattoo on his back, and I even remembered his house and bedroom.

He has aged considerably since I first saw him, but he is still attractive, with a cheeky, boyish face. He's now in his late thirties, greying, overweight and often looks flushed and sweaty (I suspect he has high blood pressure), but there's definitely something sexy about him. He's single, but as he works long hours he never gets the opportunity to meet ladies to date.

I've seen him about six times in total. This time I hadn't heard from him for over six months, after he cancelled on me at the last minute but paid me for the inconvenience. Often he wants to see me at short notice, when the stress at work gets too much. The text came through, and fortunately I was free that evening. We normally did an overnight, but this time we arranged to meet for a dinner date as I wanted to get home to my own bed because I don't sleep well when I'm with him. We usually stay at his house on the outskirts of Leicester, so we made plans to meet at 6.45p.m. at his local Indian, so that he could stay late at work.

I arrived early and was expecting him to be a bit late. I assumed he'd arrive in his Bentley, but he called and said he was just dropping off one of his business partners and that he'd be arriving in his gigantic 4x4. When he arrived, it felt like some illicit meeting of two married people, both arriving separately and meeting in the car park. Wherever we go in his village, people always want to talk to him. It's clear he is very popular and well liked, and he always introduces me to people. I feel like I'm his new girlfriend, meeting all the locals.

As soon as we entered the restaurant, the owner's son greeted us and spent quite a while chatting at our table, and then the owner came over, but eventually we were left to choose our meal. Simon was downing the wine like there was no tomorrow, so I reminded him about his car and he said he'd jump in mine and leave his. In the six months since our last date, he'd joined a dating site and met a few strange ladies. The first time he slept with one of them, she complained that he didn't cuddle her in the night, and then she got a bit obsessive and scared him off. So, he's given up on online dating and is back to booking me, which is great!

Really, he can't get his head around the whole escort thing – I can't win with him. He's extremely insecure, and knowing that he's paying for companionship knocks his confidence; he thinks I'm just putting on an act for him, because his self-esteem is so low. I constantly try to make him feel good about himself with genuine compliments – I tell him I enjoy his company and feel very relaxed with him, and that I'm attracted to him, but then I know he's thinking, 'well, why should I have to pay?' I almost think he would prefer it if I was some random woman, only interested in him for his money.

He asks why he can't have a girlfriend like me, but then says he wouldn't want to go out with an escort because he couldn't bear the thought of another man 'sticking his thingy into his woman' – which is understandable. He thinks I detach from the experience when I have sex with him, and I do, but it's subconscious. Although I find him attractive, I wouldn't want someone like him in my private life because he's selfish in the bedroom. He thinks that because he's paying, he can treat me like a prostitute, and that's why I'm not attached to him in any way – he's not trying to please me. I'm in the role of pleasing him. He's never been interested in trying to make me orgasm or giving me pleasure before he takes it for himself. I put up with it because I do genuinely like him, and his ego is very fragile. Maybe he treats me like a prostitute because it's the only way he can get his head around paying for companionship.

He mentioned that he wanted to take me to Portugal. He's been on and on about taking me away for over a year now, so I've learnt not to take these comments seriously. He asked over dinner, 'So, how much for me to take you to Portugal for a week?' but then he added, 'For me?' It annoys the hell out of me when rich people want discounts. Not particularly wealthy people rarely ask; if he wasn't well-off, I'd quote him considerably less than my usual £5,000. But as he's loaded and I'm not, I think, why should I give him a discount? I don't even think of him as a regular, seeing him once or twice a year; he shouldn't begrudge paying me. I feel I have to explain my reasoning when I tell him I won't be able to offer a discount – I shouldn't have to, but I know he won't get round to taking me away anyway, so it all seems a bit pointless.

The food was delicious, but as he was paying the bill, he pulled a small packet out of his shirt pocket. It was liquid Viagra. My heart sank. I told him it was dangerous for him to be taking it if it wasn't prescribed: many guys don't realise you need to be extremely careful and that it can be very dangerous if you have high blood pressure or heart problems. Some people have a weak heart and don't even know. It had left a blue patch, as it had leaked onto his shirt pocket. He started lapping it up from his fingers. Because I'm so comfortable with him, I can be my normal cheeky self, so I told him he had another thing coming if he thought we were going to shag for three hours! 'Let me have it!' I snapped. He passed it over and I rolled my eyes, wrapped it in a napkin and left it on our table as we left. He then said he had a raging hard on.

As we walked out, he told me to follow him. It was clear he was planning to drive, even though he'd had a bottle and a half of wine and an Irish coffee. I told him if he got into his car, I would go home. He protested that he couldn't leave it overnight because he needed it, but I wouldn't budge. Thankfully, he saw sense and got in my car. I wondered how often he drove while drunk — he claimed he never did, but I suspect it was quite often.

When we got back to his, we sat in his boys' lounge. There's a bar, a huge TV and comfy leather recliners, all with drinks holders — I can just imagine a bunch of lads watching a fight or football game there. We watched TV for about an hour before he said he was going to shower.

After a relatively short session, which ended up in him having to bring himself off while I sucked on his balls, he then said he was tired. I asked if he wanted me to leave, and he apologised and said yes. I told him it suited me too, as it meant I wouldn't get back too late, so I ended up leaving 40 minutes early.

CHAPTER 13:

The Boyfriend Experience

Recently I had the best date I've ever had with a guy. Sexually, it was everything I craved, and in fact I was concerned that I might fall for him, if I saw him regularly. I was to meet him for an extended overnight date, with a view to us travelling away together for a few days. The day before, he said he liked light coloured lingerie and stockings. I had my reservations because he'd made these requests, but he hadn't said 'I want you to wear this and this', he'd said it was what he liked, so I didn't expect he'd be the controlling type.

There's a misconception that all escorts must be real sex experts and I think many men are intimidated. I'm old-fashioned, and I love long, sensual foreplay, with lots of kissing and caressing and massage before moving on to sex. I'd like to explore tantric sex with my next partner, as I think I have lots more to learn about sex and reaching mutual sexual fulfilment.

I arrived to meet my date and my first thought was that he was very attractive. He was in his forties and I could see through his T-shirt that he had a toned, trim body. He'd bought me flowers and Swiss chocolates, and had put a card in the envelope with my fee. It was just before Christmas, and he even gave me a mince pie which his mum had made, in a little bag that he'd managed to squash. It was so sweet! He wasn't full-on, he was relaxed and we spent a good hour just chatting.

We went out to a pub I had recommended. Over dinner, he was a great companion, interesting and attentive. Back at the room, I lit candles and we put on some music. We kissed for ages – he was a lovely kisser. He didn't just try to get my clothes off, and he wasn't too eager. Eventually he undid my dress and I let it slip to the floor. I'd worn hold-ups with light-coloured lingerie, as he'd requested, and from the look in his eyes this met with his approval. Usually my lingerie comes off so quickly on dates that I wonder why I bother, but we caressed and kissed, savouring each stage of intimacy as we slowly unwrapped each other like presents. It felt as though I was with my lover – this was like a BFE (now there's a new one – a Boyfriend Experience!). *And* he was paying me. It was heaven! I started to realise how guys must feel when I offer them this kind of intimacy. It was so easy to feel something for this guy, because of his tenderness and the connection I felt we had, and for the first time I was confused. He made it all seem so natural – maybe I should suggest he becomes a male escort!

When we were both naked, he kissed me and stroked me so wonderfully gently that it was highly erotic. I was so turned on and he hadn't even begun exploring the obvious bits. I lay back and savoured every moment – I had barely touched him, but it was clear that he wanted to enjoy me first, so I let him, knowing he would reap the benefits after. Many guys go straight for the breasts and vagina/clitoris. It's so obvious. I actually like foreplay to include a lot of caressing and kissing of other areas of the body first, and I think that's why often I don't orgasm with work. If someone goes straight for my clitoris, I usually can't get turned on enough to have an orgasm. If only more men realised this!

His oral sex was perfect, soft with a featherlike touch, and I was frustrated to find that I couldn't orgasm, even though I was incredibly turned on and extremely relaxed. This may have had something to do with the time – it was getting late (for me), and I was very tired. Most escorts are nocturnal ladies of the night, but I'm one of the rare few who love daytimes, especially early mornings. After an early night at home, I love getting up at around 6a.m. in the summer when it's bright.

Much as I was enjoying myself, I was fading rapidly. I reached down to finish the job myself with my fingers, which didn't take long because he had put in all the groundwork. He then lay on his back and I stroked and kissed him, down his body and inner thighs, taking my time before licking his balls and moving my tongue up the shaft of his penis, and then I took him in my mouth. He savoured this before suggesting I get a condom. Then he turned me onto my back and slowly entered me. Instead of pumping away like a sex-crazed loon, he took his time with deep, precise, slow thrusts. It felt amazing! For the first time ever I wished we'd skipped dinner but how was I to know he wouldn't be a 'typical' client? He built himself up to climax and collapsed on top of me.

Unfortunately, I ended up not being able to make the dates for his trip so he took someone else. Part of me hoped he didn't have a good time and would choose to take me next time! Hopefully we'll meet again.

I look forward to seeing my elderly regular, John, of whom I'm extremely fond. He finds it difficult to sneak away as he still works full time and has no reason to travel. I only see him two or three times a year, when his wife goes away for long weekends with her friends. I'm pretty sure he doesn't see anyone else, and I know he would see me more often if he could. He's very respectful, and not demanding in the bedroom, which is appreciated. It's mostly about companionship, even more so with him than my usual dates.

We always have fun, and I'm quite cheeky with him, which I know he enjoys. We go back and forth with banter, and even when I'm cheeky, he laughs and tells me I'm lovely and beautiful. He'll try to stroke my leg in public, and I'll playfully push him off and tell him to behave. He loves it! As with most of my clients I don't like to be seen holding hands with him (only real couples or those in some sort of intimate relationship hold hands), and I feel self-conscious when he tries to show affection in public, but that's not because it's him, I feel that way with all the clients I see. We talk about all sorts, and age has never been a barrier as far as the conversation side of things; I think it keeps him young, having someone like me to have fun with.

Much to my surprise, he once asked if I could set him up on a date with a different escort! I got quite shirty with him and asked who he thought I was, his bloody secretary? We had a laugh about it and he ended up booking me instead. I think he respects the fact that I'm not different with him because he has money – I treat everyone the same, money or not. I'm sure there are escorts that do treat wealthy people differently, and other women that do so, too. But he doesn't fit the 'rich mould', anyway – although he's ridiculously loaded, he's not emotionally needy or tight, like many of the rich guys I meet. John doesn't spend money on himself; he even drives an old blue work van. He's extremely generous, though, and loves to shower me with expensive gifts: beautiful clothes, shoes, bags and jewellery. He says it makes him happy and I genuinely believe it does. Who am I to deprive an old man of happiness?

Our first shopping trip came about because he frequently asked me to wear a short skirt out on our dates, which I refused to do. I said I wouldn't be comfortable because of how old he was, and also because of the classy restaurants we go to.

But I offered to make a deal with him: if we went shopping together, he could buy me something and I would wear it, and it would be a compromise; something I didn't consider too short and he didn't think too long. He agreed, so I took him to a designer shop in Birmingham. I was trying to find something I could get a lot of wear out of, but he really liked a purple silk Gucci dress, which was £1,000. I wasn't sure about it, but it did grow on me. I tried it on with some black patent and gold platform heels, and he kindly bought me the shoes and a bag to match.

Since then he's taken me on numerous trips and bought me jewellery, perfume and other clothing. He once picked out a beautiful coat that was £1,500. I would have never chosen it for myself, but when I tried it on, I loved it. He has a very good eye for what suits me. Most of the dresses he buys me, he thinks are too long, but they sit on my knee!

Here's my wish list for the perfect client:

- He would have impeccable hygiene and wouldn't have skipped the shower or be washing in the sink on my arrival!

- He'd be a true gentleman and treat me like a lady, not give me room service or burger and fries on an overnight date.

- He'd take time to get to know me before moving on to more intimate moments, and not slobber all over my face as soon as I get in the room or ask for a 'quickie' when I arrive before we go down for dinner.

- He'd be friendly, genuinely interested in me as a person and interesting to talk to, rather than giving yes/no answers to avoid a proper conversation in the hope that the more quickly he answers, the sooner we'll move on to more 'fun' things. If he's funny, that's a bonus.

- He wouldn't brag or talk about himself too much. There's nothing more unattractive than someone boasting about where they've been and what they have, trying to make you feel so lucky to have been chosen for a date. I had one cancellation message that read: 'I'm sorry I have to cancel as my Bentley has blown a gasket and I can't afford to get it fixed'. Whatever!

- He would appreciate good food, wine and company. Guys spend so much money arranging a date, so when they try to scrimp on hotels and food it's really annoying. I don't want to eat at a two-for-one and have an overcooked steak with grotty chips and a £5 bottle of wine! There are plenty of inexpensive places that serve quality food, so there's no excuse!

- He would be easygoing and not rush things. An 'eager beaver' is such a turn-off! If my date's tapping his foot and summoning the waiter when I still have half a glass of wine or a mouthful of dessert, I'll make sure I take my time, just to make a point.

- He thinks it's just as important for me to have a good time, too. The guys who ask where I'd like to stay and what I'd like to eat are usually the most chilled and lovely clients, because they want me to enjoy our time as much as them. Then there's the ones who don't spend any time preparing and book a hotel next to a railway line to save a bit of money, and we end up eating at a Pizza Hut (which I do enjoy by the way, but on this occasion there was urine all over the floor in the ladies'), and on that date I didn't get a wink of sleep thanks to freight trains running all night. Of course, he got the bitch from hell in the morning!

- He would enjoy lots of foreplay and take the time to turn me on, knowing the more he puts into the experience, the more he'll get out of it.

- He'd take pleasure in giving me pleasure before having an orgasm himself. Yes, I know it's old-fashioned, but I do think that when it comes to orgasm it should be 'ladies first'. The guys that I put the most effort in with are the ones who make the effort. After all, it's a two-way street!

- Preferably, he'd be trimmed or shaved below. There really is nothing worse than pubic hair. I don't want to be flossing with men's pubes, so if they're shaved or trimmed, I'll spend much more time down below. Shaved balls look like juicy plums! Mmmm...

- He'd be a great kisser! Most guys can't kiss and I find it revolting. How on earth they get by, I've no idea – I don't want a drop of slobber on my face after I've kissed them! Why do some men try to open their mouth so wide and swallow my face, while clamping my head with their arm so I can't pull away? It's hardly surprising their wives seem prone to headaches!

Diary: February 2008

Last night, Gerry used the 'F'-word on our overnight date and I ended up putting him straight. 'Gerry,' I said, more abruptly than I intended, 'you don't really consider me a friend. When I was worried about you because I hadn't heard from you, you ignored all my correspondence and had no consideration for me whatsoever, and this time I didn't hear from you for over six months.' 'It's just how I am,' he replied. What rubbish! I can't imagine he ignored any of his proper friends.

For about four years, I saw Gerry once a month at his home in Leicester for an overnight date at his house. He's in his sixties, a bachelor lawyer, who had previously suffered from cancer. When I didn't hear for him for quite a few months I got extremely concerned, as you would with someone you cared about, who had previously been ill. So I emailed, called and even wrote to him, pleading for him to let me know he was OK, but I didn't hear from him for three months.

When we met again, he explained that three people who were close to him had died.

I empathised with him, but that's when I realised that he didn't think of me as a 'friend' because he would have responded to one of my messages if he had. He couldn't say that he hadn't realised I was worried. He did know, because I said so in all of my correspondence.

I often wonder whether any of the people who have stopped contacting me over the years have died or had bad accidents, because let's face it I wouldn't get any family members or friends informing me if they had. I genuinely care about people, especially the regulars I see, with whom I have built up a relationship of sorts, yet I'll probably never know if anything bad happens to them.

Eventually, Gerry got back into the routine of seeing me once a month, but then after Christmas last year he stopped contacting me again. I only got in touch with him when I was raising money for cancer research and wondered if he'd sponsor me, as he was a survivor himself. He said he would, but when I emailed him about the money, he ignored me again. I chased him a couple of times and then just left it: he has never given me that sponsorship money.

Out of the blue I had an email from him, enquiring about an overnight date (the one I went on last night), saying he was sorry he hadn't been in touch but he'd been ill. I felt that it was selfish of him not even to let me know, and rude of him to have ignored my emails. At least he could have sent a quick one-line email or text. I've known him nearly six years, so I believed we had some sort of friendship. Obviously not. The frustrating thing is that every time we met he constantly went on and on about how he considered us 'friends'.

All the way to my date with him, I worried because I knew I would have to say something if he used the 'F'-word, and I was pretty sure he would. On the drive to his house, I reminisced. I was looking forward to seeing him; we'd had some great dates in the past. Overnight dates with Gerry were almost as good as it gets, for work dates. When we first met, he told me he liked his own space when he slept, so asked if I minded sleeping in the spare room. I couldn't believe my luck! This was my ideal escorting date: not only my own bed, but my own room.

We were like a really old married couple with our set routine. I would get to his house at 7.30p.m., we'd have a brief chat and then head out in the car for dinner. He lives in the country, so there's lots of cosy country pubs that do fantastic food, and often we'd go to one of those. We'd have a relaxing meal before heading back to his house. Then we'd go straight up to his bed to play, before going to our separate rooms to sleep. In the morning I would get up whenever I fancied. I always stayed for a couple of hours, so it never mattered when I got up. He'd hear me get up and would make me a cup of tea, which he'd bring me in my room. We'd sit and drink tea in my bed, before having our morning fun. After building up an appetite, we'd go downstairs for breakfast before I made my way home. It was always the same, but it suited us both.

When we first met I remember he talked constantly about himself. After at least half an hour of me listening, I cut him off and asked if he'd like to know anything about me. There's no point in being subtle with guys with Single Man Syndrome: they're too self-obsessed to take hints. It's usually the reason they're single, whether they want to be or not. Most get away with their selfish behaviour because, unlike me, the majority of women will not challenge them.

Gerry, in all fairness, is unique (in my experience) because he admits he's selfish and – in his own words – 'not sufficiently interested in other people'. He apologised and was actually pleased I'd made a point of saying what I did. He told me to tell him in future if he ever talked about himself too much again. Since then he really tries to be interested in me and asks me what I've been up to, but I know he's just faking it. I could never go out with anyone so selfish in my personal life.

He'll never ask about things we've talked about in the past, whereas I'll remember things about our last date and then bring them up when I see him again. For example, if he's playing badly at golf and has had one of his tantrums on the range, on our next date I'll ask if his golf's improved. Because he isn't interested in me, he never remembers things I've talked about previously – he just asks what I've been up to. So, it's easy for me to start a conversation with him, but he never, ever tries to initiate one with me. That means we always start off talking about him, and the date last night was no different.

I initiated the conversation, and he told me all about his golf, his house and his work, and his thoughts on reality TV shows and Gordon Ramsay. Another sign of his selfishness is that he never offers me a drink when I arrive. When I have visitors to my home, the first thing I do is offer them a drink.

During the drive to the pub he eventually asked what I'd been up to. It had been a year since I'd seen him, so I didn't know what to say... where should I start? My mind went blank, so I started by saying I'd got my Brown Belt in Aikido, but when he didn't show any interest in that, I steered the conversation back to his favourite subject: him. He's known about me writing this book for a while, but he's never once asked me how it's going.

After a very tasty meal, we made our way back to his house. I opened the drawer in my room to see if he had any candles left from our previous dates – he had a whole collection that had grown over the years. He lit them and put them around his room. I had a black lace and cerise lingerie set on, and his eyes lit up when he saw me. It wasn't long before he undressed himself and we settled on the bed.

He is fascinated with my boobs and loves to spend ages playing with them. It turns me on, too, which is a bonus, so it didn't take long for my bra to be removed. We spent about an hour playing. Thankfully (and surprisingly) Gerry is not selfish in bed, so most of our bedroom time he spends pleasuring me – licking and caressing me. By the time we have sex he's usually so turned on that it doesn't take him long to come, and then we snuggle in a post-sex embrace for a short while before I go back to my room.

This morning, I stayed in bed until 9a.m. When he heard me get up, he went to make me a cup of tea, and by the time I'd had a wash and got back into bed, leaving the door open so he knew I was up, he arrived with two cups of tea. We must look like a married couple, drinking tea side by side in bed, him with his jogging bottoms and T-shirt on, me in my nightie. All I needed was the hair rollers! It's our 'moaning morning' – every morning after our date we sit in bed and whinge about the world today: the prison system, problems with plumbers, squirrels, computers, people, diet, weight… Anything we have to whinge about, we do it in the morning with a cup of tea.

Once we'd both finished our tea, I turned on my side towards him and snuggled up. He put his arm around me and then he turned to face me, too. He was grinning, so I grinned back at him with a mischievous glint in my eye. We kissed and caressed each other. Gerry always wants reassurance that I am enjoying myself, so he talks a lot during our intimacy. He'll ask things in the third person, like, 'Do you think Bea would like me to play with her boobs?' If only he could be as caring and interested out of bed!

It's always a quicker session in the mornings, and after about 30 minutes of foreplay and a short sex session beginning with me on top, and ending in missionary, he came. We embraced and carried on our chatter, before I prompted him that I needed feeding, so we showered and went downstairs for breakfast.

Before I left, he said he'd like to see me after his operation.

CHAPTER 14:

The Girlfriend Experience

Everyone has their own interpretation of the sought-after 'Girlfriend Experience' (GFE), but to most people it means a lady who makes the experience fun, enjoyable, unhurried and relaxing – more like a 'real date' than a commercial encounter. However, in practice whether this is actually achieved depends on many things, including personality, chemistry and mutual expectations.

The opposite of the GFE is the PSE (Porn Star Experience), which has a strong emphasis on the sexual side of the encounter, and as the name suggests, these girls generally offer hardcore, porn-style sex. These experiences can be cold and detached, with lots of fake moaning and no kissing, and sometimes it's clear the girls aren't really enjoying themselves and are just doing it for the money.

There are also the very sought-after ladies who have the ability to switch between both – allegedly giving a GFE in public, and a PSE behind closed doors. I personally think there's no such thing, as the two things contradict each other.

Girls offering a PSE generally don't kiss, and I can't imagine any boyfriend, no matter how much he loved wild sex, would find that acceptable. And surely guys would want real moaning and groaning, not the fake groans associated with the 'Porn Star Experience'? So, when guys say the lady offers a GFE/PSE combination, they actually mean it's a raunchy GFE – I suppose like having a girlfriend who's a nymph, and who genuinely enjoys sex.

My personal opinion is that you can't offer a GFE for any date that doesn't involve being wined and dined. It's about more than the sex – it's a total package, and I think you need to get to know someone outside of the bedroom to really have a GFE. That's why I mostly see people for overnight/dinner dates and longer. The things that I think make me a good GFE are that I am affectionate and tactile and I love kissing and intimacy. Also, I'm a friendly and warm person, who is caring and giving when treated respectfully. I'm told I can quickly put the most nervous and shy person at ease. I enjoy being wined and dined, and having weekends away. I'm well-mannered and likeable, and I don't wear a lot of make-up. I prefer the natural look, with no hair or nail extensions (only boob extensions!). I don't wear tarty, revealing clothes for my dates, and I dress like a lady. One of my clients recently told me I was the most sensual woman he'd made love to. He'd seen a number of escorts and said he felt that many of them were trying to detach themselves from the experience, but he said I made things feel very natural.

In my early days there was one time when I wasn't very professional. I was on an overnight date with one of my regulars and we'd got back to the room after dinner. I'd had a whole bottle of wine with dinner, as he was Muslim and didn't drink. When we got to the room, I was feeling quite tipsy, and sexually frustrated. I wanted him to make an effort and make me come, which was silly, and I remember saying to him that he didn't care about my enjoyment and never tried to please me. He looked quite startled at this little outburst – he'd seen me so many times, and it had never bothered me before. He left the room, and I paced around in tears and called an escort friend for advice. I couldn't drive home, and if I left it would be really awkward.

Would he see me again? While I was still on the phone, he came back in. I terminated the call and decided to apologise. After a while, I joked that he had just got the ultimate GFE – with arguments, tears and everything. No one can accuse me of not being like a real girlfriend!

Escorts specialising in offering a GFE are great at finding a connection with people and putting them at ease, but this can be misinterpreted. One of the dangers of offering the GFE is often emotions get involved (usually on the guy's side), and once they're there, this makes things extremely difficult. When I find a client I can be my cheeky, funny self with, someone who's easygoing, fun and great company, it's dangerous because they rarely last as a client. I have lost regulars that I have been genuinely fond of because they have misunderstood our connection. I'm not saying I'm a fake, but we all do it – we let different bits of our personality shine out with different people. Here's an email I received after a date:

Hi Bea-Beautiful

Thanks for a really relaxed and stimulating night.

Escorting may well be your 'job' and you are indeed clearly very 'professional' (having integrity and being organised, reliable and considered in a manner that gives your clients the experience they are seeking)...but...and I don't mean 'but' as in not acknowledging that all that is a compliment to you...but ...as in additionally...I found you such a warm and natural delicate flower, and so very easy to talk to. I am sure this must happen often with you...I found myself talking about difficult areas that I would not normally share with a companion...so thank you for being so bloody feet-on-the-ground open and normal. You are so easy to be around – ranging from hearing about you crashing your car to lying naked with you and enjoying your smile and chemistry.

You are a really lovely person. I am in danger of rambling and boring you, so just thanks and really hope to meet up again in the near future...with the thought that last night disappeared so quickly that I would hope for your company for a much longer time.

Good luck, take care...check that mirror...and look after that fierce independent streak that defines you!
Love
Max x

The main disadvantage of being a good GFE is guys falling in love. This is very flattering, but also inconvenient because the relationship has to be terminated, which is a shame because the guys who end up falling for me are usually the ones I'm also genuinely fond of.

I once saw a guy on his birthday for two nights. I had seen him previously for an overnight date and we got on really well. As a thoughtful gesture, I decided to make him a cake, which I covered in pink icing and lots of sweets. I also made him a card with a picture of Michael Caine on it, because his voice reminded me of him, and I bought him a bottle of his favourite tipple. I wasn't physically attracted to him, but we just clicked and we had such a laugh together. I was so comfortable with him that I even did girly trumps at his request! We were in fits of giggles. He kept saying that surely I didn't act like that with everyone I met, which was true, but it didn't mean I wanted to be with him. After all I didn't really know him; I'd only met him twice.

He knew my dad had a shop in Derbyshire as he was a sales rep and covered the same area. So, after our date he sent a massive bunch of flowers to the shop. He admitted that he had fallen for me and asked if we could take things further. I declined as I didn't feel the same way about him and was disappointed when he said he couldn't see me any more.

This also happened more recently when I lost a very special client friend. The first time I saw him, we met for a three hours in his hotel room. He was an attractive guy in his fifties, but he looked much younger, with a kind, smiling face. He was in the IT business and was divorced. We got on really well. He was surprised to find that people actually took me away for a few days at a time and even went 'out' with me. I found it most amusing and joked with him about why he would find it so hard to believe people took me out and about. I said I didn't think I was bad enough to have to be hidden away! He said that when he'd previously met an escort, he had asked if she wanted to go to the bar for a few drinks, but she had preferred to stay in the room. Maybe it was a hotel in her local area and she didn't want to be recognised, but personally I love to be taken out and shown off!

So, there and then we arranged a five-hour dinner date for a couple of months later. I really enjoyed his company and thought that as he was so easygoing and undemanding, I would want to see him regularly. Our fifth date was a couple of nights in Venice in January. We had a wonderful couple of nights in the Danieli, a beautiful old palace converted into a hotel. The first day there, we enjoyed afternoon tea in the dining room. It was very cold and miserable, and I found I didn't want to really go very far from the hotel, but he was fine with this and went off to do his own thing. We had a trip in a gondola, which I had always wanted to do, and enjoyed wonderful meals at a couple of restaurants.

We grew very fond of each other and I genuinely looked forward to our dates. Because of this, I gave him my real name to make a booking to Vegas and I didn't take the full deposit from him. I also sometimes booked and arranged hotels for us as I knew he was busy, and I would arrive early so I could spend more time with him.

The last couple of times I saw him, he had made certain comments that made me think he was getting too attached. He would constantly flatter me, saying how beautiful I was. This was lovely at first, but then it got a bit too much. The last time I saw him, I suggested a couple of drinks in the hotel bar after dinner, which we didn't normally do. It was 12.30p.m. before we got to the room, but because he was usually so quick to please in the bedroom, I wasn't too concerned. However, when we got there, he decided that, for the first time in the two years I had known him, he was going to give me oral sex. This was pretty pointless as it was so late and I just wanted to get to bed! If I'd known he was going to do that, then I would have gone straight to the room when we got back. After a while I finished the job and came, then sorted him out. He said in a half-serious, half-joking way that he would have to stop seeing me because it was getting too much, and that I was so beautiful.

When I sleep with someone I always face away from them, because I hate the thought of them peering at me in my sleep. It makes me feel very vulnerable. This was something that never concerned me with him, because he always made me feel very comfortable. However, he then confessed that he liked to watch me as I slept, which really freaked me out. After this date, I decided I needed to be tactful to try and salvage things, because I knew we were on a slippery slope. I decided to email him and just let him know that I was a little uncomfortable about some of the things he had said, and to say that I couldn't offer him anything other than what we had: a professional relationship. I then explained that I enjoyed his friendship, and was genuinely very fond of him, and I did my best to flatter him with genuine compliments, so I didn't offend him.

Our next date was due about three weeks later, and I was supposed to be booking the hotel. I didn't hear from him, so I emailed again. It took him two weeks to get back to me, which as we had a date coming up was extremely frustrating. He said he felt awkward that he had made me feel uncomfortable (I noted there was no apology for this), and that although he had never seen our relationship as anything but professional, we should have a 'break'. I tried to save the connection with a couple more emails, but to no avail. He mentioned three times that he felt awkward for making me feel uncomfortable, but he didn't ever apologise, which I found rude and very odd.

There are constantly threads on sites like Captain 69 about guys falling in love with escorts. I know of a couple of situations where girls have had successful relationships with people they have met through work, but I think, mostly, it doesn't work out. Usually the guys are married and going through a mid-life crisis. Either that, or they're single and looking for a girlfriend, and then they would usually expect you to stop escorting.

I once read on a forum someone referring to the Girlfriend Experience as 'a crap shag, no come in mouth and fake emotions!' First, I know GFEs who do offer CIM (Come In Mouth). But second, how does one define a 'crap shag'? For me, a GFE is a two-way, mutually enjoyable experience, but a Porn Star Experience (PSE) is something I interpret as a one-way experience, with the lady entertaining the guy. With a GFE, the more you put into the experience, the more you get out of it, so one can only assume any guy who says the escort is a 'crap shag' is also one himself.

When I first started escorting I learnt the hard way about boundaries between escorts and friends. When guys want to be your 'friend', they tend to offer to help you out with things so they have an excuse to keep in contact with you. Not long after I began, there was a guy I had seen twice before. On the third occasion, after dinner, he took me to the gay village in Manchester. I was really quite tipsy as we'd had drinks with dinner and then had more drinks afterwards. By the time I got back to the hotel, it was really late and I was tired, so I ended up going to sleep, much to his disappointment, and promised to make things up to him in the morning. After that, he kept in touch by email, and offered to help me build a website. He once came to the house and spent time helping me with my computer; he took a disk of my photos and said he would create a website for me.

He never did anything about the website, but he emailed me every day and I replied. After a couple of months' communication, without him booking me, I told him that he would have to stop emailing me and that I just didn't have the time to email every day, seeing how he hadn't booked me for a long time. He wanted to be 'friends'. He panicked and tried to call me, but I ignored his calls. Then he frantically started emailing me, saying he wanted to sort things out, but as far as I was concerned there was nothing to sort. Eventually he gave up, but he wrote me a spiteful review on Punternet, under a different name, which was the total opposite of the glowing report he'd previously given me. Fortunately, the website's owners could see it was from the same guy and so it was deleted.

Things also got messy with my solicitor friend. He often travelled a good three hours to come and help me with buying my apartment. It wasn't really necessary for him to travel to see me, but he did so because he enjoyed spending time with me, and I too enjoyed his company. On one occasion he said he would come to the open evening of the apartment block, and said that as it was going to be finishing late he'd have to stay over, implying I would be staying with him. I understood what he was saying, which was that he was expecting to sleep with me. When we checked into his hotel, I was relieved to see there were twin beds, but he wasn't so happy about it. I explained to him how I felt, and eventually he understood. We had crossed the escort/friend boundaries, mixing business with friendship, and I lost him.

One of my friends has actually booked me as an escort before. Yes, I know you shouldn't mix business with pleasure. It's a grey area for me because my business *is* pleasure, but as one would expect, from that moment on, our friendship was pretty well doomed! My friend Nat and I used to go clubbing in Doncaster many years ago, and we met a couple of guys there, Luke and Nas. I had a brief fling with Luke, and Nat was seeing Nas, but it only lasted a few months. Years later, for some strange reason, I got a call from Nas and we became friends. I didn't see him very often, but occasionally he would take me out for lunch; I spoke to him almost every week, but probably saw him maybe a couple of times a year. He was young, good looking and loaded, but I was never interested in him sexually as he wasn't my type.

When I started escorting he asked about my fees and said he would book me. I thought it might be a bit weird, but he was an attractive guy and I did know him, so I decided it would be OK. He had previously booked one of my escort friends and paid for her to stay overnight, but when he called me I was disappointed to find he wanted to see me for a couple of hours only. Normally, I wouldn't go to Doncaster for two hours, but I made an exception because I knew him.

I arrived at his house, and we got a takeaway and had a chat. He told me he had a girlfriend, who he loved. Yeah, right, that's why he'd booked me! It did seem very surreal, as we had known each other for such a long time. After about an hour, he put on some porn and wanted us to get down to sex. He wanted porn-style sex, and that's not what I offer. I didn't enjoy the experience at all; it was the most fake job I have ever been on. He couldn't come and thankfully I ended up leaving early, at his request.

We still stayed friends, but he spent a lot of time out of the country so we didn't speak to each other quite so often. After about a year he called again and asked me to visit him for a couple of hours. I really should have declined, but I didn't. On my way there, he called and told me he didn't want to talk when I arrived – he just wanted sex. That's not what I offer or advertise. He was one of those people who doesn't realise that every lady is different and that while some sell sex, others offer companionship. I told him I wouldn't turn up on any two-hour job and jump straight into bed, and I wasn't about to make an exception. He made me feel like a cheap whore and I ended up in tears, so I turned around and made my way home.

A few months passed and he eventually called to apologise, but then asked if he could book me again. I told him no, that I wouldn't see him again for any amount of money. I didn't like the way he treated me with so much disrespect.

I have a lot of guys that I meet through work wanting to be 'friends'. Once I saw a guy for an overnight in Manchester. At the time, I was using a driver who'd pick me up and take me to meet my dates. Johnny, my date, said that he had never booked an escort before. Guys always say that, even though they have seen other ladies. I think they're hoping to get special treatment. He was a small, average looking guy, and we were about the same age. We ate out in a restaurant I had chosen, where we had a lovely meal with champagne. It transpired we knew some of the same people, too – he knew guys in the year above me at school. Back at the hotel, I suggested a bath. We had a gorgeous suite with a lounge and bathroom downstairs, and a bedroom upstairs with a free-standing bath. I lit candles and put on some music.

Johnny didn't seem very comfortable with the whole 'escort' experience. He appeared nervous and on edge (in retrospect it could have been drugs), and I don't know why he booked me in the first place. We had a bit of a kiss in the bath and moved on to the bed, but he suddenly said he couldn't do it and when

I asked what he meant, he said, 'This.' I said we didn't have to do anything he didn't want to do, and told him he was paying for my time, not sex, so he shouldn't feel bad. I wanted him to be comfortable, but I don't think anything I said or did would have made a difference. We chatted, and he said he wanted us to be friends and that he wished we had met in different circumstances. I wouldn't normally agree, but I thought we got on really well, and as we knew the same people I agreed that we could try and be friends. After chatting for a couple of hours, eventually we went to sleep.

In the morning my driver, Pete, was waiting for me and we still hadn't had breakfast, so we invited him in to join us. This was very surreal – we were all sat having tea in the morning, Pete, Johnny and me! I did keep in touch with Johnny, but I knew I wouldn't be able to see him very often. I have quite a few friends who live far away and I don't get to see them as often as I would like, and it would take me a good three and a half hours to get to where he lived, so it did seem a bit pointless. However, he invited me to a corporate hospitality do with his business partners and their girlfriends. He picked me up from Manchester, and on the way to the party he told me that I'd have to lie to his friends about what I did, because he thought they'd think he was paying me. I hadn't really thought about it before, but assumed that as we were now friends, I would just be honest with people. I wasn't happy when I thought of all the lying I would have to do, and I felt very uncomfortable with the whole situation. I knew then it would be unlikely that we would be good friends because he was uncomfortable with my job.

During the meal, I was asked questions about how I knew Johnny and what I did for a living. I told them I sold things on eBay and did a bit of modelling. I don't think any of his friends or partners would have had a problem with how we had met – the only person with a problem was him! He was a nice guy, but I do think he has 'issues'. Really, he should have been looking at dating sites, not escort sites. I suspect that he was a serial escort user, and I think he freaked out with me when he realised we knew the same people.

Sometimes guys with no intention of ever making a booking try to waste my time with emails and phone calls, wanting to be friends. They tell me all about themselves and ask if we can get to know each other, but when I give them information about my escort services, they act all offended at the suggestion that they should pay to see me, and say they just want to exchange emails and 'get to know me'. I don't have time for that and it's not what I offer! Then there's Tim, a guy who has been stalking me with texts. I replied once because I thought it was someone I knew. When I realised my mistake, I ignored him. He's since sent me a couple of emails and about 14 text messages, with no intention of actually booking me. He wanted to meet up with me socially for free, watch me have one of my photo shoots, and then pay me for any time spent having sex. How insulting can someone be? Another guy I'd seen once years ago contacted me, and I said we should meet up – obviously as a booking, seeing as I'm an escort. This was his response:

'I would love to meet you again. Are you talking about as a client or just as friends? I have not seen an escort for several years. Would you consider wearing a very short micro mini skirt with no underwear underneath?'

Er… no! I hate it when people waste my time like that.

A guy from Captain 69, who I introduced to escorting, also tried to cross the escort-friend boundary. We met for an overnight and I was his first 'escort date'; I remember he bought me quite a few gifts. Shortly after that, I went off to New Zealand for a couple of months. On my return he contacted me, wanting to meet up again and telling me all about the women he'd seen while I was away, which I thought was damn rude. I told him I wasn't interested in his conquests – I wasn't about to tell him about all the sex I'd had, or the men I'd seen. He said he'd taken to having a bit of sex before dinner on his dates with other escorts and wondered if I would oblige, even though he knew from meeting me previously that this wasn't the way I did things.

I spend a lot of time preparing for my dates, and the last thing I'm going to do is jump straight into bed and get sweaty. I want my dates to be like real dates, to a certain extent at least. Therefore, I told him that I would only meet him if we went out for dinner first. He agreed, and again bought me some very extravagant gifts, which was very kind, but I knew he was trying to buy friendship. Sure enough, he said he wanted us to be 'friends'. I never saw him again as a client. He tried to meet up with me socially whenever he was in Nottingham, but it was clear he didn't want to pay for my time, so I haven't seen him since. He sees escorts maybe a couple of times, then tries to be their 'friend', buys them gifts and takes them away instead of paying for dates. I'm not interested in that kind of 'friendship.' As I said, I like to keep things separate. He says he has numerous 'escort friends', but if he has to buy gifts all the time to keep them or help them with their websites, then they're not true friends.

Diary: January 2008

'Is it business or pleasure?' asked my nosy taxi driver. Both, I thought, but answered 'Pleasure.' 'I have a date,' I offered. 'Well, I hope he's paying your cab fare,' he said. Yeah – and the rest, I thought!

I arrived at the hotel, about twenty minutes from where I lived, five minutes early for my 7p.m. dinner date. I knew the hotel layout, so I headed straight for the lifts. My date, Geoff, answered the door in his shorts and T-shirt. His iPod was playing softly in the room. I've seen Geoff about six times: he's married with two older kids, and he's slightly overweight with a shaved head. He's quite good looking, but he's so full on, it's mentally exhausting!

I settled myself down in a chair and we immediately started talking about his holiday. He'd been to Africa over Christmas and New Year with his family and his kids' partners. 'Did you get the text I sent you Christmas Day?' he enquired. 'Yes,' I answered. I hadn't replied to it. 'Did you get the one I sent at New Year?' he continued. 'Yes, but I was busy with friends and family,' I offered, both to explain my lack of response and also to suggest he should have been doing the same.

He told me in November that he was going to text me at Christmas. This is what I mean when I say he's full-on; he's trying to get something emotionally from me, and I'm not going to give it. I have no interest in getting involved with him – this is my work, not my personal life. He shouldn't be text messaging me – Christmas is a time for family and close friends, and he should save his emotions for his wife and family. He said he wanted me to know he was thinking about me, but what was he expecting me to say? That I was thinking about him too? He's obsessed with talking about how he sees me as a friend and how special I am to him. It's annoying, and I feel suffocated by him sometimes, but he's a lovely guy when he's not talking about 'us'.

He'll email at length about how much he appreciates me, looks forward to our dates and sees me as a friend. I ignore all the emotional talk in his emails and only reply to send him information about our dates, but he still carries on. It makes me feel uncomfortable because the feeling's not mutual. I'd feel closer to him if he never mentioned anything, but because he's always trying to get more from me emotionally and to make me feel guilty when I don't reply, it makes me feel like I don't want to see him at all.

Once I left him at a hotel to get a cab home and he said, 'Text me when you get back or I won't sleep.' I told him I was extremely tired and I might forget, but not to worry as my regular taxi company would be dropping me at my door and watching me get inside safely.

Again, he said that he wouldn't sleep, putting more pressure on me! Don't get me wrong, I appreciate the fact that he cares, but it's not like I'd be waiting out on the street for a cab, or having to walk anywhere in the dark, or even using a cab company I didn't know.

Anyway, back to our date. I steered the conversation away from us, and back to him, his family and their holiday. He asked about my Christmas and New Year. After about an hour chatting, he got changed and we went down to dinner. We spent the next two and half hours eating and talking – I really enjoy his company when he's not full-on. After polishing off our three courses, we made our way towards the exit for the bill. As we were standing there, he was getting so close that I could see he wanted to lean in for a kiss. I don't do kissing in public, and he was looking at me expectantly and hesitantly, obviously not wanting to make a fool of himself. It was like he was telepathically trying to send the message to me to kiss him. I ignored it, and he soon signed the bill and paid, so we left for the room.

I left him tinkering with his iPod while I went to the bathroom to change. I was wearing hold-ups, a net camisole, a thong and high heels. When I came out, he was naked and in bed; the room was lit by soft candlelight, with Sinatra playing softly in the background. Perfect. 'Wow!' he said, as I approached the bed. Sexily, I crawled over, kissing him gently on the lips and moving on to a lingering French kiss. It didn't take him long to slide down one of my camisole straps to access my breast. He complimented my assets while sucking urgently and taking my other strap down. I let him enjoy my breasts before lowering myself down onto his body, kissing softly down his torso before taking him in my mouth. He stroked my hair and I looked up at him from under it, knowing he was watching. 'Let me lick you,' he murmured, turning me onto my back and pulling down my panties. I love his technique – it's like he's lapping at a saucer of milk! He then moved up to kiss me, and I grabbed his member and started rubbing the end on my wet clit.

'Do you like my cock on your clit?' he enquired, obviously keen to talk dirty. 'Yes, I love the feel of your hard cock on my wet clit, it feels so good,' I replied, matching his terminology, while stifling a giggle (I find dirty talk cheesy when I'm working). 'Just use it, use my cock to make you come!' I knew that wasn't going to happen because I couldn't quite get the angle right, so I reached for my trusty vibrator and finished the job. Wet and horny, I then went down on him again before grabbing a condom and slipping it on. I climbed on top of him and thrust him inside me. I was grinding up and down for a few minutes before he started panting and it was clear he was about to come. I looked him in the eyes while moving my body up and down on him. He shuddered to orgasm and I collapsed on top of him.

But then he started talking about 'us', and saying that I was the most sensual woman he had ever been with in his whole life. Geez! He was telling me that he loved spending time with me and that I meant such a lot to him, that he saw me as a 'special friend'. He told me he thought about me every day. I felt sorry for his wife and I wondered if he was like that with her. Eager to stop that conversation (again), I quickly offered to dispose of the condom and climbed off him, slipping it off to take to the bathroom. We had around half an hour until my taxi was booked, but he's so full-on after sex that it's almost as if we haven't done anything and he's starting foreplay all over again!

He went in the bathroom after me and I quickly put my lingerie back on because even after we've had sex, he wants to constantly grope, stroke and kiss me. I can't bear it! After I've had sex, even in my personal life, I like to just lie, cuddle and stroke, with the odd lazy kiss. He came out of the bathroom and lay next to me. Sure enough, he tried to grope my boob and I knew he wanted to carry on with full-on French kissing. It made me feel queasy and I tried to cover my breasts with my hand. Shortly afterwards, thankfully, he got up and said he wanted to show me something on his phone. He showed me his dog and then a picture of his wife! 'Can you see now why I like long hair?' he asked. What an odd thing to say! 'No,' I said. 'That's my wife and she has long hair.' Unbelievable! Had he no shame? She was beautiful.

I didn't feel guilty as I don't know her: he should be the one feeling guilty, but I'm always surprised how many married men can see escorts and not feel guilt. I try not to think about it too much. Sometimes there are genuine guys who have valid reasons for seeing escorts, perhaps they don't get sex or intimacy from their wives; other times, they just want to play the field. I don't know what his personal situation is – he hasn't mentioned a lack of intimacy from his wife, so I don't know; but if he's as full-on with her as he is with me, I wouldn't be surprised if she avoided sex with him! Maybe she's pleased he's not pestering her for sex if he's seeing escorts – that's sometimes the case. However, what does amaze me is the number of women who assume that their husbands will accept having no intimacy in their marriage and won't go looking for sex elsewhere.

It was time to go, so I gathered my belongings and said my goodbyes. He said it would be a couple of months before he next had an opportunity for us to meet, so I told him I'd see him then, thanked him for a lovely evening, pecked him goodbye and left. Fortunately my taxi was waiting, so off I went. To prove a point, I didn't text him when I got home!

CHAPTER 15:

A Couple More Great Guys

From: Jetlag
Location: Nottingham
Notes: Formerly worked as Barbie of Derby and Miss B
Date: 16 Nov 2002
Day of the Week: Friday
Time of Day: N/A
Type of Visit: Outcall
Time Spent: 4 Days
Price: 4,100, including flights
Place: 5-star hotel
Description: B is a beautiful, perfectly shaped blonde, who's sensual and great fun. She has an engaging, caring personality.
Comments: I vowed I would never write a review of any escorts, especially those who had given immense pleasure. I changed my mind with Bea – on reflection, I don't feel it is right not to share a gem. This was my third time with Bea in the last few months and it has been both a privilege

and pleasure to get to know Miss B. I believe I now know what makes her tick! She is a delight to be with – in my case, twice in England and once in Hong Kong. She's sensitive, beautiful, enchanting and all in all, a deliciously sexy lady. You can be proud to take her anywhere and despite her young age she can converse on a wide range of subjects. Immediately you will forget, as I did, that she is an escort and not someone who you have known for years. Her 'GFE' is as genuine as it comes. This is not because she is an excellent actress, but because she is genuine to the core. So much so that, as you would expect from a real girlfriend, she will soon let you know if you have been a complete klutz! (Ouch! That's my hair you're pulling!) But rather than diminish the quality of the encounter, this added to it. As with all those who have reviewed her previously, I am not going into any graphic details here, but suffice to say she will transport you to heaven and back if you push her buttons and you treat her with the respect she so richly deserves. You have to be warned! Bea leaves a vacuum behind her when you say goodbye. I will certainly be churning out the widgets at a faster rate to be able to continue to enjoy her company and pleasure-giving, which leaves me with an immense sense of well-being. Recommended: Yes. Would You Return: Yes.

Some of the nicest guys I've met have not been memorable for the sex, but because they are such amazing people. I met an incredible guy the other week. He wanted to arrange a platonic, last-minute date in Leicester. In a situation where there's no hotel reservation, I usually need to be paid upfront into my bank account. As this was so last-minute he wasn't able to transfer the money in time, so I had to make a decision on whether he was genuine based on speaking to him. My gut feeling told me he was, and I didn't have any other plans, so I

A Couple More Great Guys

decided to go. He wanted to meet me for three hours at a shopping centre. He had a stutter and said he used a walking stick, and he didn't sound very old.

I arrived in Leicester and called him once I'd parked up, but I was concerned when I got his answer phone. Waiting in my car, I felt very vulnerable and started to wonder if it was a wind-up, or if he was watching me from somewhere. After waiting nearly half an hour, I paid for my car parking and left. He then rang me to say he'd had a bit of a fall. I was a bit annoyed because I couldn't understand why it had taken him so long to call me, but I told him I'd go back to the car park and find somewhere for us to meet. I then had to wait another 30 minutes before he called to say that he was in Pizza Express.

I found my way there, and as I went up the escalators I saw the restaurant and smiled at an attractive guy in the window who looked uncannily like my ex, James. It turned out he was my date! We decided we'd try and find somewhere where we could get a hot drink, so we left the restaurant and stopped on a bench in the shopping centre while he fumbled about to give me my cash which was all crumpled in his pocket. I hoped there weren't any CCTV cameras on us!

I was amazed to find that he was so independent, even though he was quite severely disabled. He couldn't lift either of his feet off the ground as they were both turned inwards, and he had to use all his concentration to shuffle one foot in front of the other. Immediately, I realised how difficult it would be for him if he fell, and I felt bad for being annoyed earlier; he didn't have the use of one of his arms, either.

We found a Starbucks that was close by, and I went in to get us coffee and cakes. He was such a lovely guy, and I realised how much I took for granted; he enjoyed films and worked from home. If it was such an effort for me to walk, I couldn't imagine what I'd do. It had taken him half an hour to get from one side of the shopping centre to the other – I had so much admiration for his sheer determination.

I had never met anyone with a real stutter before so I wasn't quite sure what to do. So, I sat and waited patiently for him to ask questions, and when he was on the last word and couldn't get it out, I thought, what do I do? I'd wait a few minutes, thinking, should I just answer the question because I know what he's going to say, or should I say the last word for him? Would that be irritating? He kept saying sorry when he couldn't get his words out, so I wanted to help him, but wasn't sure what to do. So, I varied it – sometimes I waited for ages and let him finish, sometimes I said the last word and sometimes I answered the question; I didn't want him to feel uncomfortable. He complimented me, but mentioned that now that I'd met him, I probably wouldn't see him again. I told him he was wrong and that I'd be honoured to be invited to see him again. He was thrilled – I think he thought I'd be embarrassed to be with him, but I wasn't. I know of many escorts who are embarrassed to be seen out and about with guys who are old, disabled or big. Some are shallow and only want to be seen with flashy, young business guys.

We arranged there and then that we would meet and go to the cinema the very next day; we met at Birmingham to catch the train together, and when we got on the train he had to lie down on the floor and shuffle into the carriage. I sat on the floor with him, trying to make him feel more comfortable. When he got off the train, he had to shuffle across the platform and try to launch himself up onto one of the benches to then attempt to stand. There were people looking at me, wondering why I wasn't helping him. I told him to tell me if there was anything I could do to make things easier – I had tried to lift him, but he was a dead weight and I felt I was just getting in the way. I think he was too proud to want to be helped and he probably knew from experience it was easier to do things himself.

It took us half an hour to get to the cinema complex, which was across the road from the station. First, we went to Pizza

Hut to grab some food. Our table was up some steps, so he asked me to put a chair by the steps to help him get up. He then moved from chair to floor to the table. I really enjoyed his company, and we then went to the cinema. We enjoyed a romantic comedy before leaving to catch our train. It was very difficult for him to get out of his seat and steady himself back onto his walking stick, and I was worried we wouldn't catch the train, but he was sure he could make it. So, we began our slow walk back. I was worried he might fall down the slight hill, so I tried to keep him steady. He kept apologising for struggling, but I said he had nothing to apologise for; I told him I was sorry he had to struggle. I left him in Birmingham, where I had to sprint for my train. I'm not sure if he will call again, but I thought he was one of the most amazing people I had met.

As an escort you have to learn to read the signs and work out what people want. In my early days, I met a guy for an overnight at his home in Sheffield. We went out for a leisurely dinner and he told me how he was struggling with women today. Like most men who are single at 40, they're not sure where to go to look for dates, so he ended up going to nightclubs. He'd meet ladies and ask them back to his place for a coffee. The thing is, he really did mean *just* coffee, and he was shocked when women would think he was trying it on. They'd try to initiate sex and he wasn't comfortable with it. He went on about it so much that I got the impression he was hinting he didn't want me to jump on him! So, we spent a lovely evening together, just socialising, and the next morning we said our goodbyes.

A year later, I heard from him and he thanked me for my patience the last time we met and said that this time he was ready to go all the way. Some escorts don't read the signs and will jump on a guy as soon as they walk in the door. Obviously, some men love this, but many find it bloody scary! I never jump on anyone when I arrive and I make it clear that

I'm not that type of escort. The common misconception is that men who see escorts only want sex, but as you've already seen, this isn't always the case. Offering the GFE means I often spend long weekends away with my dates, and I've had some amazing experiences.

Diary: September 2008

Today I met my regular, Jack, who's an accountant. He's extremely overweight, but very sweet, polite and softly spoken.

We'd arranged a back-to-front dinner date (which I wouldn't normally do) as he had to be out of his hotel room at 12; I couldn't meet the day before for a dinner date. So, we met at 11a.m. for four hours. This would mean one hour in the room, then going out for lunch for the rest of the time.

I wasn't quite sure what we'd do in the room. When I first met Jack, I tried to be intimate with him, but he wouldn't do a thing to me and he'd just hold my hand in place if I was touching him down below and pant and groan, so I had to train him. As soon as he clamped my hand, I moved it away.

I used to give him oral sex, but I'd be dressed and he wouldn't even get hard, so it seemed pretty pointless and I've never made him come. Then, because he's a really bad snorer and a restless sleeper, we have separate rooms on an overnight. Yup, it's the WFE – Wife Experience!

We meet about twice a year and he keeps coming back, though, so I must be doing something right. I'm pretty sure he enjoys my company as much as I enjoy his. When I arrived, I wanted at least ten minutes to settle in, if we were about to get frisky, so after a couple of minutes I asked if I could have a cuppa. As he made it, I sat on the bed, in case he did want some bedroom fun. However, once the tea was made, he sat in a chair. We chatted away, but he clearly couldn't relax because he said he was hungry. He also said that he hadn't slept as it was so hot, and he was extremely tired. Eventually I moved to sit near him.

Over 30 minutes had gone by and he was clearly happy enough, just chatting. I did ask a couple of times what he wanted to do, but he just said he wanted to go and get food, so eventually that's what we did. I certainly wasn't going to jump on him! If I'd had any inkling that he wanted to get intimate, I would have made a move but there was nothing.

Then I excused myself to go to the loo and I noticed he hadn't even showered: the shower was bone-dry and the towels were in place, apart from a crumpled hand towel on the floor. He's probably been washing his pits in the sink, I thought – yes, he's another single man! There was also no soap open, so I knew he hadn't washed his hands after he'd been to the toilet. So many men don't, and it's really quite disgusting. He also has been known to wear the same tight boxers that he's slept in overnight, two days running. I was quite glad I hadn't made a move!

So, we both gathered our things and he gave me my fee, then out we went for lunch. Usually, we eat at the same local restaurant. Thankfully, it wasn't busy – he has awful table manners, though he's been getting slightly better with my guidance. Maybe I should charge extra and offer etiquette lessons for manners and hygiene? He always talks about dieting and exercise, but every time we meet he's the same weight. When choosing his food you can guarantee at least two courses will be unhealthy. He thinks he's being healthy by sacrificing the bread, but then he has belly pork, a fish dish (ooh, well done him!) and then ice cream to follow. I really don't mind what people eat, but first, he's always talking about diet and exercise when clearly he doesn't do enough of either. And second, he eats with his mouth open, constantly.

I've taught him not to speak with a mouthful of food, but I now need to work on teaching him to eat quietly because it really puts me off. Although he's a single guy, he doesn't really suffer from SMS but he lets himself down with the poor table manners and hygiene. He's such a lovely and genuine guy, though, and when he's not eating noisily, I really enjoy his company.

While we were in the restaurant I saw a guy leering over at me and I wondered what he must have thought. We look an odd couple, but I guess we could be business partners or acquaintances. I know many escorts don't like to be seen with guys, if they're not flash businessmen, but it really doesn't bother me – if they eat like a pig, it's themselves they're embarrassing, not me.

Even before our time was up, Jack was ready to leave. He didn't have to get back to work, so part of me was a little insulted that he wanted to get away, but on the other hand it's refreshing that he's not clingy and trying to take advantage by keeping me longer. I think it was purely the fact that we'd both had enough to eat and drink, so it was time to go.

As we left the restaurant, I gave him a hug and was about to give him a kiss on the cheek when he sneakily swivelled around and got me bang on the lips. Flustered, I looked around to see who was looking... fortunately I didn't see anyone I knew!

CHAPTER 16:

The Dreaded Question

'So what do you do?' – it's the dreaded question.

I get various reactions when I tell people what I do for a living. Some are totally shocked, because to them 'escort' equals 'prostitute', and although I've nothing against anyone prostituting themselves, I probably wouldn't be so honest about what I did if *all* I did was sell my body. The fact is, people pay for me as a package – a 'girlfriend' and companion for an evening out or a few days away. But because some people think it's all the same, I can see them thinking 'have you no shame?' The looks of disappointment I get anger me – there's nothing worse or more patronising than them thinking or saying 'You could do so much better for yourself'. To me, it shows how judgemental some people are; they know nothing about how I run my business.

Others are intrigued and ask all sorts of questions. I don't mind them asking because I like to educate people, and give them a better understanding of how I work and what my job is about.

My family all know what I do. My mum and dad accept my job, which is pretty cool, but they still don't like it. I don't think many parents would be that understanding, though. Dad used to go on about the 'abnormal world' I live in, but he is semi-retired and never really does anything or goes out; he doesn't have a network of friends. It's my mum that's like me – a 'get-up-and-go' person with a large social circle. So, to me, *his* life is 'abnormal'.

Dad's a very intelligent man but if it wasn't for Mum, he wouldn't socialise at all! He never calls anyone on the phone; in fact, he has never called me or my siblings, ever. I sometimes find him incredibly hard work! Recently, he has changed his view a little since I treated him to a Genesis concert this year and took him on a balloon ride (which a client had paid for, but it was cancelled due to the weather). Lately, he's been saying that I've done so much, far more than many others my age, and that I've had some wonderful opportunities. I'm glad he understands my lifestyle a little more now.

Dad still has his little digs, though. I took my parents and grandparents to see *The Lion King* in London, and I laughed at my dad, who arrived at the station with a packed breakfast, packed dinner and a flask of coffee! I'd booked us in for a three course brunch at 12, so why he even needed breakfast I've no idea. He then tried to say, 'Well, we can't *all* afford to buy expensive sandwiches,' which was a dig at me, saying I was extravagant to even think such a thing. How ridiculous! If Mum was on her own she'd have pushed the boat out and bought something to eat if she wanted. The silly thing was that she made him leave his rucksack at St Pancras and that cost him £6.50, so it would have been cheaper for him to buy those 'expensive' sandwiches!

I'm extremely interested in psychology and I often try to analyse myself and others. I'm also curious about why I made the choice to escort. Being a very sensitive, emotional and affectionate person (I think this is what makes me different from my parents and siblings) I remember craving attention from my dad from an early age – he keeps his feelings and emotions all tucked up. As a child I worshipped him. I used to love it when he played guitar and sang to us. My favourite was 'Dream', a 60s classic song. It would nearly make me cry with happiness and I just wished he would do it every night.

I often ran away. I remember being so upset once that I took my rabbit down to the woods and wandered around aimlessly. After about an hour I was bored, so reluctantly I made my way home. My dad found me at the bottom of the drive and asked where I'd been. Teary-eyed I informed him I had run away. He laughed and said, 'Well, you're back now, so get inside. Your mother and I are going out, and you're babysitting.' I was gutted! 'Yes...but I *ran away*, you know'...I pleaded for him to take me seriously. He carried on laughing (but not in a nasty way), as he repeated that he'd heard me the first time. His way to deal with emotional things was to make a lighthearted joke out of them.

My dad chased me across the park once, and that's when I got him to say he loved me. It's the only time he ever has. I was running off for some reason...I guess I was about 13. I didn't want to have to create dramas to get a reaction from him; I just wanted him to be affectionate towards me. He wasn't affectionate to my mum either – she'd sit on his knee and he would look at us kids and pull a face. We thought it was hilarious, because he was such a joker, but I realise now that he struggles to show affection to anyone.

More recently, my dad refused to help advise me about buying my apartment because he thought it was ridiculous that I was spending so much money. After a number of conversations with my grandma (my dad's mum, who I was very close to) she finally got him to speak to me and he did help me, even commenting to the solicitor that he thought it was a good investment, although he had never said anything positive to me about buying it. My grandma told me that my dad loved me very much and said that although she knew he didn't say it, he was also very proud of me. I wonder if, deep down, getting positive attention from older men on my work dates is in some way a substitute for the affection I crave from my dad.

Despite our troubles, I have a lot of respect for my parents because neither of them has tried to get me to change my job. They know from experience that it would be pointless, and I'll always do what I want to do, anyway. None of my siblings has their own property and a successful business. I had bought my place and was running my own business by the time I was 25, so although I'm the only one without a degree, I know my parents are proud of what I've achieved. Occasionally they will tell me that I've done well for myself, and I know that I have.

My brothers are uncomfortable when people ask what their sister does. They both feel embarrassed. I once went to my brother Andy's work do, and one guy asked what I did. My brother just glared at me, giving me that 'Don't you dare tell him!' look – which I ignored – and he made a real fuss about it. Sometimes he tries to act posh, so he wouldn't find it acceptable to have a sister who was an escort. Recently, one of his friends asked me why I didn't speak the same as him – I told him we all went to the same school, but my brother fakes his posh accent. He thought it was hilarious! On the other hand, one of his friends' mums once asked me if I was a hooker. I said no, wondering why she'd used that derogatory term, before correcting her and saying that I was actually an escort. It transpired my brother thought it would be funny to tell her I was a hooker. I told him I'd remember that, and next time any of his friends asked what I did for a living, I'd say I was a hooker.

My mum's friend Margaret found out what I did recently. Margaret has known me and my family for years, and although she's a bit older than Mum, she is very open-minded. I have always been very fond of her, but I wasn't sure how she would react when I told her what I did for a living. When I explained to her about my job, she thought it was extremely exciting and told me I was very lucky to have such wonderful opportunities for travel. If I join a new group, I don't tend to tell people, because I don't want them to gossip. I may, however, tell a few people I think I can trust as I get to know them.

No matter how many times I'm asked what I do for a living, I never get used to it. My mind starts whirring and I have to decide in a nanosecond... am I going to tell the truth? If I decide to lie, I go for my standard response – 'I sell on eBay' – while praying that'll be the end of it, but it rarely is. 'What do you sell?' they ask. 'Do you make good money from it?' I have sold bits and bobs on eBay, but I can't go into too much detail in case I'm asked questions that I'm unable to answer. But the alternative is to tell the truth and have people think 'hooker'. Why do they immediately think 'escort' means 'hooker'? It's like they lose the ability to hear anything after that. That one little word leaves my mouth and suddenly a whole host of ideas enters their minds.

Yes, I enjoy sex and I've been told I'm good at it, but I'm not a nymphomaniac. I wish I was – I could make a fortune! I have no interest in other people's boyfriends, unless they pay me for their time – only joking! Girls, I'm not out to steal your boyfriends. Finally, I'm not easy. I don't sleep around outside my work. In the last seven years, I've had three long-term boyfriends and six one-night stands; that's all. Also, I'm not filthy rich: my rates mean I can earn a lot, but I can be without work for weeks at a time, and as I've said before, my expenses are extremely high.

Being a very honest and open person it troubles me to lie, which is why most of the time I tell the truth. The only problem with the truth is that there's no grey area in some people's eyes. They think all men pay escorts just for sex, but that's not the case. Someone once paid me £100 just to sit outside a bar with him and talk to him for 40 minutes. He just wanted people he didn't know to see me with him.

Generally, I'm very honest about what I do, because I don't feel it's anything to be embarrassed about. I love my job, and I'm good at it. Sometimes there are people I wish I hadn't told – once they know, they act completely differently around me and don't know what to do. It shouldn't matter what I do, and I get frustrated sometimes when people judge me; the way I see it, lots of people have sex with colleagues, so what's the big deal? OK, so I might do it more often, but so what? I know there are single women who sleep with more men than I do!

I think a lot of women are wary and feel intimidated by me, which I find sad because I'm a very honest, open, generous and loyal friend. Because of people's attitudes, often I've struggled to make and keep friends. Escorting can be a very lonely profession, even more so for those leading double lives. Not working in an office environment means I don't have local 'work' friends. I work from home on my computer and I go out on dates.

It's not as if I haven't tried to make local friends – I joined the gym and met one girl, but she moved away shortly after we met. I joined the scuba group and found myself a boyfriend, but didn't make lasting friendships. I go to salsa classes, but haven't met anyone there who has become a friend. Then I joined Aikido and it's only there, after two years, that I've met a couple of people I keep in touch with. I also met two amazing friends a year ago by chance, through a friend of a girl I know from work, I used to see them at least once a week but both of them are now settled into relationships so unfortunately I don't see them as often as I'd like.

A lot of Matlock people now live in Nottingham but there's only one reliable friend, Katie, who I keep in touch with and go out with. Most of my close friends live dotted about in various places around the country – Liverpool, Manchester, London, Leicester, Matlock and Chesterfield.

Once, I went to collect a book a neighbour had borrowed, and her partner looked like a rabbit in headlights as he opened the door. I didn't want, or expect, to be invited in; I just wanted to collect my book. He started stuttering about how he was busy working and couldn't invite me in; it was bizarre. Then my neighbour called that evening and was suspicious, asking why I hadn't waited for her to get back from work before collecting my book! It was most odd, and I can only think it was because of my job. Some guys that I know socially will often act differently around me when they're with their partners. This can be frustrating – they look uncomfortable and it makes them look like they've done something wrong! Some just ignore me if they're with their girlfriends; it's almost as if they expect their girlfriends to have a problem with them speaking to me.

Some of my close friends seem obsessed with having some sort of male interest in their life, which I find quite sad. Maybe I'm just a bit odd? Probably I'd be celibate if I wasn't working as an escort – I'm too busy trying to sort my life out to worry about men, and I'm not someone who needs a partner to complete me. I think it's extremely important to be happy with myself. Don't get me wrong, I would love to find Mr Right, but I'm not going to go out looking for him. I just get on with my life and if it's meant to be, I'm sure our paths will cross.

I also find people think that I lead a different lifestyle from the one I actually live. My uncle's new wife cracked a joke about me not knowing how to use a vacuum cleaner because she assumes I'm wealthy and no longer do my own cleaning. If only! Once, when I was planning a trip to my uncle's farm, I found a company that hired out tents, and for an extra £20 they would deliver it, put it up and take it down. As the weather was supposed to be bad, and I hadn't camped for years, that sounded great. Everyone teased me about being too posh to put up my own tent, and joked it would be a mansion with people feeding me grapes!

The thing is, I shop in Asda because it's cheaper than Sainsbury's, and Primark because it's less pricey than Topshop; like everyone else, I watch my pennies. I'm not saying I never buy anything designer, but the majority of my wardrobe isn't exclusive: like most people I love grabbing a bargain. Most of my designer gear John buys me.

Earlier this year, I went to meet one of my friends, Laura. We ended up meeting her boyfriend in the pub. It was St Patrick's Day and the place was heaving. A couple of guys stood up so that we could have seats, and then Laura stood up to talk to her boyfriend, so I was left talking to his friend, which I didn't mind. Then a guy I knew from years ago plonked himself next to me, Timmy. He's late thirties, but looks older. He used to be quite attractive, but he has a huge nose that has been broken a few times and he slicks his dark blond hair back with Brylcreem. It's not a good look. Unfortunately, he sparked up a conversation that went like this:

Him: So what are you doing with your body nowadays?

Me: What do you mean, 'with my body'?

Him: Last time I saw you, you were in a top-shelf magazine, legs akimbo.

Me: That was a long time ago. I'm working as an escort now.

Him: Oh, you're still doing that? So how much would it cost for me to spend the night with you?

Me: I'm not going to tell you, it's none of your business.

Him: Well, I might want to book you.

Me: I'm not working right now.

Him: OK, but how much would it cost?

Me: I'm not telling you – I don't ask you how much you earn.

Him: Come on, how much then?

Me: I wouldn't sleep with you even if you paid me, so it's irrelevant.

Him: Oh, you think you're so clever!

At that point he was shouting, 'Football Face, Football Face!' at the top of his voice, just as the bullies used to do. It seemed like loads of people were looking at us, but no one said anything to him. I was so annoyed with myself for even talking to him in the first place. That's one of the downsides of being honest about my job – some people seem to think that just because I'm an escort, they can treat me like that.

I have to educate new friends about my profession because often they think that when I'm not out on dates, I have nothing to do. In fact, there's always something. If I'm not working, I'm trying to get work, and if I'm at home during the week I'll be on my computer until about 12p.m. Then I go to Aikido, and maybe do some food shopping or any other essential bits and pieces, before going back to my computer until about 6p.m. I'll cook my tea, and then if I'm having a night in, I'll watch some TV and be in bed by 9 or 10p.m; I relish early nights. I have badminton on a Monday and occasionally go to salsa on Wednesdays, and I try to keep my weekends free to catch up with family and friends.

If I'm working away for a night, it can take two days out of my week, which is a big chunk of time. I rarely do social things during the day. Friends will often want to meet up if they have a day off, and I do see them very occasionally, but knowing how my body clock works, I know I concentrate best during the day before I start to tire, so I prefer to meet friends in the evening and use my days for work.

Friends and clients often say that I must be extremely confident to do what I do. Yes, I am, but I'm sure any woman being paid for companionship would gain confidence. My confidence has grown so much because of my job. I don't feel nervous because people know what to expect of me and they know what I look like, so I don't worry they'll be disappointed. Having people pay to see me is great for my ego, especially when they choose to book me again and again. I wish, though, that I could be as confident when I meet men I like outside work.

Like most people, I'm confident in some areas but not in others. Put me on my own in a room full of strangers and I feel very nervous. I'm not good at talking to people I don't know, because I'm never sure if they'll want to talk to me. For my job, it's one-on-one, and I know people have chosen to spend time with me, which makes me feel confident in myself. A close male friend, who understands about being self-employed, frequently tells me I have to take all the work I can get. What he doesn't understand is that the reason I have been so successful in this profession and have kept a good reputation is that I'm very selective. I know he doesn't understand why I turn work down. He thinks I'm crazy, especially when he knows I need the money, but I have to keep my self respect intact, and the only way I can do that is by doing things my way and only taking on dates when I feel my client and I will be compatible. This means I'll be treated with respect and will be able to offer the sort of experience the guy is looking for. You have to have a very good head on your shoulders to survive in this business.

For example, I always make it clear that on an overnight date I like to start the evening with dinner out, not room service and I ask if that is the kind of thing they have in mind when they initially enquire. If a guy said he wanted room service or to jump into bed before dinner, I wouldn't agree to see him – I'm not comfortable with either scenario, so it means I'm not suited to these people. When girls start compromising themselves, that's when they lose their self respect. In some cases, they even end up hating men and some turn to drink or drugs to get through their work. It's a downward spiral. But I can go on my dates and not touch a drop of alcohol – I often drive to my dinner dates, anyway. I feel that guys who will agree to wine and dine me are likely to be proper gentlemen, but I do realise this isn't suitable for everyone's budget. That's why I often do special offers on lunch or dinner dates.

Diary: April 2008

'I've got a special on at the moment and a three-hour date is the same rate as two hours: £350.'

This was the text I sent last night to my date, hoping he would change our short, two-hour meeting to include dinner, one of my favourite types of date. Thankfully he agreed.

I travelled out to a hotel I hadn't been to before. I waltzed in, nodding at the lady behind the desk, and strode on towards the stairs. Up I went, but realised I was surrounded by meeting rooms. Hastily, I called my date. 'I'm lost!' I whispered. He then apologised and informed me he was in an outbuilding. So, back I went, tail between my legs, past the lady at Reception, trying to look as confident as I'd been when I breezed in!

Alan, my date, was a friendly Irish man, about six feet tall, with a full head of dark hair; I would say he was in his fifties. He'd come to Retford on business and seemed quite flustered. Apparently, there was a petrol shortage (news to me), which might leave him stuck for a few days. Rather him than me!

He wanted to go straight out for dinner, which was fine, but he hadn't given me my fee. Usually I ask, but it's always awkward. This time I decided to wait until we got back from dinner and if he didn't offer it, then I would have to ask for it.

I'd never done a three-hour dinner date before and thought it might be a bit rushed, so I knew I'd have to keep half an eye on the time. I assumed he'd be in a rush and would also be watching the clock, but he was really lovely and very chilled. We had a drink in the bar before perusing the menu. He mentioned his wife and said that he might need to make a call. I remember thinking, how can someone so nice be cheating on his wife? He seemed so genuine. We spoke about his kids, his teenage daughter's and my job. He said he thought it was a dangerous job, but I said I thought pissed-up women shagging around in town at the weekend are in more danger. He'd never considered this before, but he agreed.

Alan didn't seem concerned about the time, and we enjoyed our meal. He even asked for the dessert menu, which surprised me as I'd assumed he'd be desperate to get to the room. Neither of us ordered one, but we did have coffee. By the time we went to the room, around 45 minutes were left. I hoped he wasn't going to be one of those that took forever to come, who tried to take the piss and get me to stay longer. In the room, he went to the bathroom to call his wife and I asked if we could get the money out of the way. He apologised and gave it to me. I lit my candles and went to freshen up when he came out the bathroom.

We kissed and caressed, before rather quickly removing our clothes. I went down on him, he went down on me and, as he knelt between my legs, grabbing at my breasts, it was clear he wanted to enter me, so I reached over for a condom. It was only a few minutes before he came and we lay next to one another in a comfortable, post-sex embrace. He then confided in me that he hadn't had sex for 2 years. His wife was going through an early menopause and refused to take any medication, and he found it difficult to cope with the lack of affection or physical contact. I could tell he was slightly uncomfortable talking about it, but he said her personality had changed and she refused to talk to him about how she felt. I felt guilty for thinking badly of him cheating on his wife earlier, because I totally understood his need for affection and intimacy. How can she possibly think he's going to accept a life with no intimacy?

CHAPTER 17:

The Wife Experience

There's one regular with whom I have all sorts of exciting experiences. Single and in his forties, I'm very fond of him and he's very patient with me. The first time we were due to go away for a longer booking we planned to visit the Lake District. He asked me what I wanted to do, and I didn't know – I imagined it would be all walking, and I wasn't particularly looking forward to it because my dodgy knees limit the amount of walking I can do.

Then I decided it would be in my best interests to find things to keep us entertained, so I started browsing the Internet and found lots of sites with various outdoor activities, which I mailed through to him. He was thrilled, so I suggested an itinerary that included a sailing lesson, quad biking, rifle shooting and spa treatments. I also looked into restaurants. He was really impressed with it all and booked everything for us; we had an amazing few days. Unfortunately, I found he was a really bad snorer and fidgety in bed. Being a light sleeper I was constantly disturbed, but he very kindly offered to sleep on the sofa!

The next time we went away, I suggested Stapleford Park, a wonderful old country-house hotel. Again, I suggested the itinerary: spa treatments, horse riding, archery, off-roading in Land Rovers and a hot-air balloon ride. Unfortunately, they don't have twin rooms at Stapleford, so he booked the top suite. I ended up like a Queen, with a curtained boudoir upstairs, while he was downstairs on a fold-out bed! I could still hear him snoring, though. Personally, I'd have looked at other hotels – there must be plenty that would offer two rooms for the price of that suite, or he could even have booked two rooms at Stapleford so we could both have a comfortable night's sleep.

I look forward to our dates because he's very easy to get on with, and he's happy to go with the flow. I know it must sound like I'm not easygoing at all. I wish I was someone who could sleep any time, anywhere and with anyone! But unfortunately I can't. My mum taught me to be a very considerate person and I'm always quiet as a mouse when others are sleeping, because I hope they'll return the favour. When they don't, I find it irritating. I don't even flush the loo or put the light on in the night – I guess perhaps in that way I'm not really cut out for this escorting malarkey!

I know many people will be wondering how guys put up with me, but my good points must out weigh the bad, hence why they put up with my idiosyncrasies – which are mainly to do with my struggle to sleep. I know I'm not everyone's cup of tea, but I get a lot of repeat business and I do have regulars that I've seen for years who accept and respect me for the person I am.

Diary: July 2008

So, what do I think about when I'm on the way to a date with a person I've never met before, and who I'm about to get intimate with by the end of the night? I rewound the thoughts in my head, which ranged from thinking about the pile of washing I had to do, to what I was going to do at the weekend. Various random thoughts, like many people have, I imagine, on their way to an average day at work. None about what my date would look like or what he would be like as a person; no nerves or worries, nor was there excitement or anticipation, because I wasn't even thinking about the date.

The only time I started thinking 'work-related thoughts' was when I wondered if I might be a few minutes late. With the works on the M1, I hadn't made good time. Fortunately I breezed into the hotel a minute before my arrival time and managed to jump into the lift just as the doors were closing. There was a guy already there and, apologising for holding him up, I looked down and saw my bag was gaping open, revealing candles and vaginal lubricant. Lifts are awkward at the best of times – that uncomfortable silence when you don't know where to look. I tried to discreetly close my bag, but it's a Chloé (a gift from a client) and not the easiest of bags to close, so I just tried to hold it under my arm to squash it together and hoped nothing popped out!

I'd turned a hotel-room booking into a dinner date by offering four hours for the price of three; I wouldn't have gone for a three-hour date in the room. If he hadn't accepted my offer, I'd have offered to see him for two hours. He agreed to dinner, but when I discovered he'd booked our table for 7.15p.m., I thought he might be an eager beaver, wanting dinner to be over as quickly as possible so we could move onto the fun stuff. I knew the food there was quite nice, so I had no intention of rushing, no matter how hard he tried!

When I knocked on the door and my date answered, he wasn't as I'd imagined him to be from his voice. He was older, shorter and much larger. Not that this was a problem, he just wasn't what I was expecting. I think we all have images in our head when we're meeting someone we have only spoken to on the phone. Very bubbly and friendly, immediately, I liked him. He worked in insurance, and we spent about ten minutes talking about his job, but it was clear he would just talk and talk without offering me a drink. It's usually nerves that make people forget to offer, so subtly I suggested going to the bar for a drink and we made our way downstairs.

Immediately we started exchanging a bit of banter and I felt very comfortable as I love little take-the-piss digs. It's what a lot of real couples do, and it shows two people are really comfortable with each other. After ordering our drinks, we sat down to carry on the conversation. He was really lovely, and didn't seem to suffer SMS even though I was pretty sure he was single; he was from Essex and suggested I go there to visit him, which I don't think he would have done if he'd been married.

We got to our table 15 minutes late. As we walked into the restaurant, me swinging my hips, we passed four tables with men solemnly eating on their own all facing our way, and I wondered if any of them recognised me, or if they were envious of my dinner date. I contemplated table-hopping, like speed dating, giving each of them five minutes as a 'try before you buy' for another time! Dates can be great advertising for me. If anyone has seen my website, but hasn't been sure whether to book me and then they happen to see me in the flesh on a date, this may prompt them to give me a call another time. On dates, I've had calls from people staying at the same hotel who have spotted me on my way in, asking if I can go and see them afterwards! I never do as I am always ready for bed after work and I don't like the idea of jumping from one man to the other. I just don't operate like that as I like to know in advance what appointments I have.

We spent the next two hours eating and chatting. He was fun and I found I could be myself more than I could with some other guys. I think it's a great build-up to intimacy, foreplay of a sort, I guess, to have dinner and build up a connection with someone before you move on to an intimate level. If I just stay in a room with a guy I can't relax enough, no matter how much we chat, when the bed is there looming in the background as a reminder of what's ultimately expected of me.

He seemed to be getting a bit impatient when my dessert took a while to arrive, and then as soon as I'd finished my last mouthful, he was calling for the bill. My heart sank – this is where someone switches from being a lovely guy to an 'eager beaver', just wanting to get his rocks off. It's usually these guys who don't really care about pleasing me. I started thinking how the rest of our time together would drag, because I knew bedroom time would be all about him and I guessed that he would be selfish in bed. You might think I was overreacting, but it comes from vast experience.

Back in the room, it seemed I was right. Barely had I kissed him before he was trying to take my top off. I don't enjoy it when men want to rush things – it's a massive turn-off; I like to start with lots of kissing and caressing before any clothes come off. As I've said before, I offer my companionship, not just my body, and guys should respect that, not try to rush me. We had plenty of time there wasn't any need to rush.

Within minutes he had, with one hand, expertly and discreetly unhooked my bra. I could tell he thought he was really clever. Shortly afterwards, I was almost totally naked. I knew this side of the meeting would be a big disappointment. He was, as I had predicted, one of those guys who just waits for me to entertain him. He kept saying, 'I'm just going to lie here.' Fine, I thought, but if you do, I will too. Where are the guys who like to savour and enjoy a woman? He barely touched me, giving me about two minutes of oral sex before he tried to pull me on top of him. I think it's so rude to pull someone about – it makes me feel like a rag doll, not a person. I kept looking over his shoulder at my watch, willing the time away, but it dragged.

He was close to coming when I was giving him oral sex, and then he straddled me and wanted to slide his penis in between my breasts.

After a few seconds, he said he'd have to stop: he was about to come. I thought, get on with it! I told him truthfully that it turned me on when men came on my boobs; that was all the prompting he needed.

He went and fetched a wet towel to clean up the mess, and then we lay and chatted for the last 15 minutes or so. He said I wasn't his first dinner date, but it was the first time he'd felt so comfortable. Well, so had I over dinner – it was just a shame the bedroom side of things hadn't matched up. We said our goodbyes and he made it clear he'd like to see me again, so I obviously did something right!

As I left the hotel, I switched on my phone to receive a text from a guy called Ed, and a voicemail from him too, saying I'd been recommended by a friend and he wanted a late visit at the same hotel I'd just been to. That old chestnut! I'd obviously been spotted, and I wondered if he was one of the lonely guys I'd seen at dinner. I was tempted for just a second, but it was 11p.m. and my bed was calling.

CHAPTER 18:

So, Why Do Men See Escorts?

Women today are so independent that I think some men struggle to work out their purpose and place in the family; they don't get the reassurance they need. Women can get so wrapped up with family life, or with their job, there's often a lack of communication that leaves both parties frustrated. Being natural communicators, women find it easy to sit and talk to friends and colleagues about their unhappy home life, but men won't.

Many of the men I see are very insecure and lack confidence. One guy I met asked me if he should shave his beard off, change his hair and have plastic surgery on his face! When they come to see me, I'm like a breath of fresh air: I'm nothing to do with their home life, family or friends, and they feel that they can open up to me. I'm a bit like a girlfriend, friend and therapist all rolled into one, and they leave a date with me feeling de-stressed and much happier.

I am sure there are some women who subconsciously know their husband or partner is seeing an escort or having an affair, but they choose to turn a blind eye. Suddenly he's coming home from work happier, he's looking after himself a bit better and he's not pressurising them for sex, which eases the tension and makes home life more bearable. Guys often tell me they're 'happily married'. This either means they're delusional and trying to convince themselves, or they're happy with most of their marriage, but there's little or no physical relationship. This doesn't necessarily just mean sex – it can also mean kissing and general physical closeness.

I was sad to hear one guy tell me that his wife wouldn't even let him put his arm round her in bed. And remember John, whose wife moved to the spare room and only came to him when she wanted sex? He wanted me to stay overnight so that he could share a bed with someone. I don't even cuddle up in the night, but he just liked knowing I was there.

An elderly guy I met recently for a dinner date had been married for 45 years and had never cheated. He had also never received oral sex from his wife and she wouldn't let him give her oral sex, so he'd never done that either. He was thrilled that I would let him give me oral sex and eager to learn how to do it. It's surprising how many stories I hear about women avoiding the physical side of their relationship. Do they really expect their husbands will just accept that the sex and intimacy is gone? Ladies, it will never happen! You need to listen to your men. If you don't try to sort out your problems, guys will either book escorts, prostitutes, or sleep around and/or have affairs. Generally men, though they may accept a relationship with no sex, can't commit themselves to a life without it.

I once saw a guy whose wife had ME. She knew he was seeing an escort, he even said it was her idea. It was very surreal because she kept calling him, and he told her about me on the phone! In her situation, I would have been jealous and I'm sure she was, but wouldn't hearing all about me just make it worse? It was bizarre. We were on an overnight date and had been out for dinner. She must have called about four times –

once, when I'd just arrived, when she asked what I was like (I was half-expecting him to hand me the phone!), once after dinner, then after we'd had sex, and then first thing in the morning! I wouldn't want to know when my husband was with an escort; if I was in that situation, I'd want him to be discreet. This poor lady tortured herself, and it made me feel incredibly uncomfortable.

Many women don't want to give their men oral sex, but they're happy to receive it. Come on, ladies, no wonder these guys look elsewhere for entertainment! If you've not given your guy a blow job in the last month, I suggest you do so tonight!

The ones I feel most uncomfortable with are the guys who think they're being clever by seeing escorts, who almost brag about their infidelity. It's not big, and it's not clever, and I think sometimes they forget that I'm a woman, too.

Being someone who says what I think, I find it very difficult to keep my mouth shut in that sort of situation. I don't mind if people discreetly go and make a call to their wife, but once, when I first started escorting and I wasn't my assertive self, I had to take a pizza into the bathroom to eat while the guy made a call to his wife in the room. How rude is that? Why he couldn't have gone into the bathroom himself, I've no idea. Other times, guys don't even leave the room – they call their wives while looking at me and winking. It makes me want to slap them round the face or kick them in the balls! 'I'm just having an early night, darling'... Wink, wink.

I had one guy excitedly telling me about all his lies. Apparently he'd said he was in Manchester watching football when we were actually in London. He called his wife when we were out, and he looked at me with this cheeky face and winked as he said, 'Yes, I'm on my way to the football now.' Throughout the whole conversation he kept looking at me, smiling and winking. I just looked away, making it clear I wasn't amused, because I couldn't believe what he was doing.

That morning he told me how he'd have to check the weather in Manchester, and he'd have to find out who'd scored goals and whether there'd been any penalties. He eagerly told me all of this while I lay in bed. I bit my tongue and tried to contain my anger. He said, 'Oh, I'll stop now – I can see I'm boring you.' 'Yes,' I said, in a bored tone, my eyes still closed. He thought he was so clever. I hope he eventually gets caught out.

Another time I'd been booked for a lunch date in Newcastle. After we dined in the hotel, we went to the room for a couple of hours. It was Valentine's Day and he told me he'd be going back to the same hotel room that evening, with his wife. What a prick! He even rang the hotel when we were out to ask if they could change the towels and put a bottle of champagne on ice for later! That guy was definitely having a mid-life crisis. His poor wife!

Although I know men love suspenders, and I do think they look very sexy, I don't enjoy wearing them because they're so damn uncomfortable, so I don't keep any as part of my lingerie collection. I told one guy I'd seen before that if he bought me some suspenders, I would bring some stockings and wear them for him. When we met, he pulled out this tatty suspender belt. I held it up distastefully, and enquired where it was from. 'Janet Reger,' he claimed. Unbelievable! 'Really?' I asked again. 'Yes,' he reiterated. 'And it's new, is it? You bought it especially for me to wear?' I asked, wondering if he'd continue his obvious lies. 'Yes,' he said, 'I thought you'd like it.' I couldn't believe what I was hearing. 'Since when has Janet Reger been using safety pins to keep her lingerie together? This tatty thing has come from your wife's underwear drawer, hasn't it? Please tell me you didn't buy her this tatty old thing, because it looks like you got it from a cheap market stall!' I threw it in the bin and told him it was no good for anyone.

Would you believe there are some guys who avoid penetrative sex because they actually convince themselves they're not cheating if they don't go that far? That's what Bill

Clinton maintained, isn't it? Most men have double standards. They think it's OK to see escorts and don't believe it's classed as cheating, but of course they wouldn't want their wives to see a male escort, and they mostly believe their women wouldn't have the nerve to do such a thing. They assume that if their wives won't have sex with them, they wouldn't want sex with anyone at all. It doesn't occur to them that perhaps they're simply no longer physically attracted to them. Generally, I think women have to be stimulated mentally before they can be stimulated physically, so if they're not 'getting along' with their husband or partner, they won't feel like having sex.

There are lots of reasons why men see escorts, but over the years I've begun to notice patterns. A few years ago, as a bit of a laugh, I decided to come up with some categories for my clients and now, after each date I try and work out which group they fall into. This is what I've come up with so far. Does any of it sound familiar? First, I divide my guys into three age categories: 18–30, 30–40 and over-40s. Then, by analysing the sneaky (or sometimes not quite so sneaky) little clues they give away, I try and work out what kind of person they are and what kind of job they do. Read on:

18–30

(a) Guys looking for no-strings sex and companionship. They tend to be single guys, who are young and experienced, or guys who are a bit geeky and unsociable, or who have no confidence with women. Sometimes they're virgins, looking for someone to guide them through it for the first time. My 26-year-old virgin, Charly, is a good example: a really sweet guy, but he was totally shitting himself.

(b) Arrogant guys who get a buzz out of the fact that they can hire people for sex. They may be single, married or have girlfriends, but consider themselves a bit of a player. They tend

253

to be rich and successful, always super-confident. They don't struggle to find women to sleep with them, but they get off on paying for it and the fact it's 100 per cent no-strings attached. My friend Nas is a classic example.

(c) Clingy guys who are looking for a girlfriend and believe their paid date with an escort might blossom into a genuine relationship. They are nearly always single and usually get way too attached. Remember the guys who email me to ask tons of questions, but then get offended when I explain that I am looking for clients, not friends? Nightmare!

30–40

(a) Guys who get a bit lonely at home, who enjoy having a regular lady to see. They tend to be married and are often happy in their marriage, but have decided to see escorts because they don't feel they get enough attention from their wife.

(b) Guys who have had a bit of a mid-life crisis and need something to pick them up and make them feel attractive again. Often they use lots of different escorts. They get a real buzz from believing that someone really enjoys having sex with them, but they tend to become a bit obsessed with it all and get addicted to the review sites. These guys refer to seeing escorts as their 'hobby'.

(c) Guys who are really busy and don't have time to socialise. They are always single and normally pretty damn wealthy. A lot of them are good catches, but they don't want the complications that you get with a normal relationship. Remember sexy Simon with his Bentley? When I first met him (before he let himself go), I'd have considered paying him for a bit of time!

(d) The older breed of single guy, looking for a girlfriend. Some can be very sweet – like my Harry Potter date – but again, you have to watch out, as they can sometimes get a bit obsessed.

(e) Older, single guys lacking confidence. You tend to get fewer of these in this age group (most people have lost their virginity by the time they hit 30!). Believe me, they do exist, though. These guys are normally a pleasure to date. Remember the amazing guy I met who couldn't walk and had a stutter?

Over-40s

(a) Guys who like to be seen with attractive ladies. It's a strange phenomenon, but a lot of them get a real kick out of it, even if it is only complete strangers who see them. Guys like this have often been divorced and tend to have one regular lady. Twice-divorced Gerry is a prime example.

(b) Older guys who need a bit of a pick-me-up. Like the similar, younger group of men, they get a buzz from seeing a variety of women and are really addicted to the fantasy of being with an escort. They make up a large proportion of the forum and review sites – escorting can be a strange, surreal world, you know.

(c) Guys seeking a bit of companionship and affection because their wives refuse to give it to them at home. They have been married for a very long time and love their wives, but there's no intimacy. Women can be strange creatures: suddenly they'll decide they're not interested in love and affection, and they expect their husbands to be happy with this. It's not always sex that the guys crave, often they just long to hug and kiss their wives. Sometimes men stay in a loveless marriage because of the financial costs involved in getting divorced, and obviously some couples decide to stay together for their children.

(d) Guys who like the idea of being with a young, sexy woman. They are always obsessed with my body – one guy just couldn't stop groping my breasts and going on about my tight bum. They simply love the fact that a hot young woman is spending time with them. Again, they tend to get wrapped up in the whole escort package – writing on forums, reviewing girls, having their say in chat rooms... Remember the guy who bragged about all the 'hot' conquests he'd had while I was away?

Diary: August 2008

I rely on AA.com to get me to any destinations I don't know. Everyone asks why I don't get satellite navigation. Well, there are many reasons. First, I really don't like driving anyway. Second, I hate technology (only because I don't understand it and haven't the patience for it). And third, would I rather spend £200 on a piece of technology or a pair of designer shoes? The shoes win, hands down. Also, because of my knees, it's uncomfortable to drive for longer than about an hour, so I mostly catch the train.

The hotel I went to last night, I hadn't been to before. AA.com told me it would take me 19 minutes, so I allowed half an hour. I was meeting Richard for a two-hour date. He left me a voicemail a couple of days ago, asking me to call him back at 11am, so I did, on the dot! He was quite impressed by that, but I'm always punctual. When we made the arrangement, I asked if I should call him on my way, as I didn't want him to worry that I wouldn't turn up. 'No, I shall be as nervous as hell!' he exclaimed, and added, 'Just turn up, it'll be fine.'

When people don't mention what they'd like me to wear and we're not going out of the room, I always go smart/casual, so last night I wore a knee-length flowery sunflower-print skirt, a black gypsy top and some black heels, for a summer look. I was following my directions to the letter, but after 20 minutes or so, I realised I was heading into town the back way. We were due to meet at eight, and I really wanted to be on time, especially after him being so impressed with me calling him on the dot. Little did I know, he was having a nightmare of his own and was worrying that I'd be on time because he wanted me to be late!

I pulled over and called him to explain that I was lost, apologised and said I'd be late. Then I called the hotel for better directions and set off again. I was only about ten minutes away, so would be ten minutes late, but I hate being even one minute late, honestly! Ideally I like to be ten minutes early.

When I arrived, it took me a while to find a parking space. He'd left clear instructions on how to get to the room, as it was one of those hotels where you have to walk for miles once inside the building. I'd forgotten the room number and so I called him again: '501, is it?' 'No, 510!' He sounded panicked. I finally found it; phew, what a palaver! Richard had a warm, friendly face, glasses, a little short moustache and lots of tattoos on his forearms, but his dress was smart. I would say he was in his late fifties, early sixties. He offered me a glass of wine from the bottle he'd brought with him.

He was really lovely and sweet – even though there was a two-seater sofa, he perched on the bed. This gave us a bit of space and certainly made me feel more comfortable. He was very nervous, and then

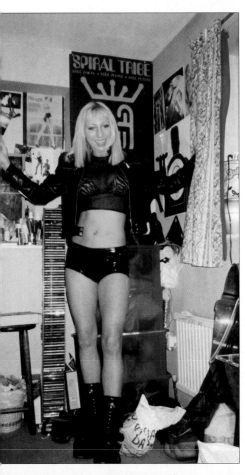

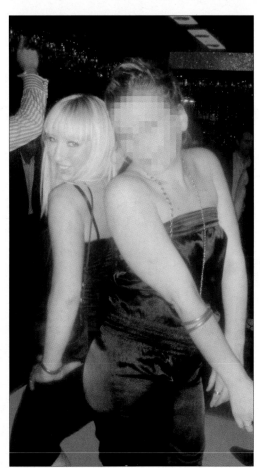

Above left: Ready for a night on the tiles! This was after I started escorting, so I'd have been 25.

Above right: At the Empire Casino opening, Leicester Square, with my friend Nat.

Left: Nat and me raving it up at Tribal Gathering 2004.

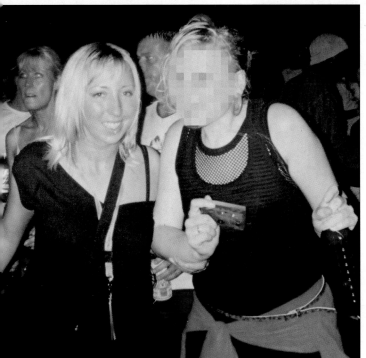

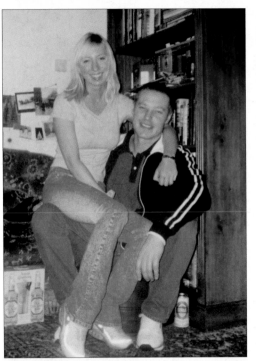
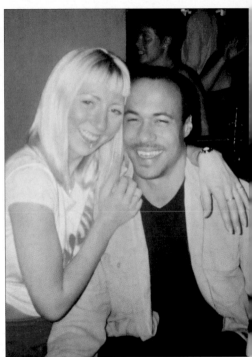
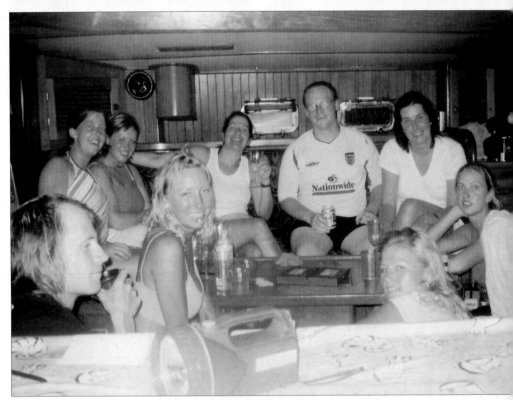

Above left: Me with Alex at my mum's for our first Christmas together.

Above right: With Kenny at a club in Nottingham.

Below: Australia 2005 – a hairy experience on a boat in a tropical cyclone, believe it or not!

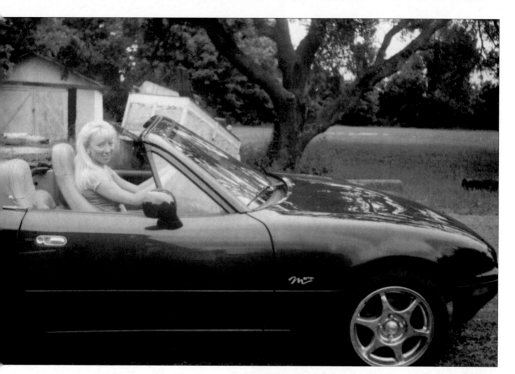

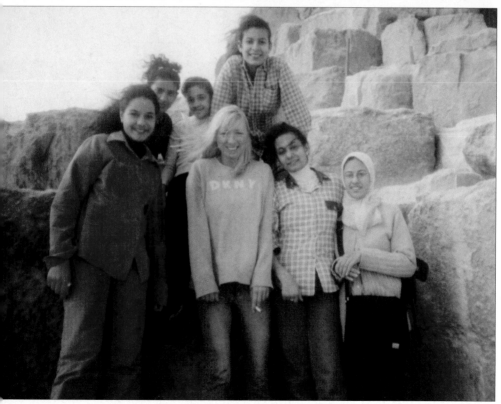

bove: Michael's MG before I crashed it… whoops!

elow: On a work date in Egypt – my date took me to the pyramids. It was my first job
ut of the country.

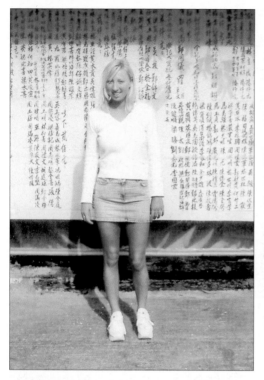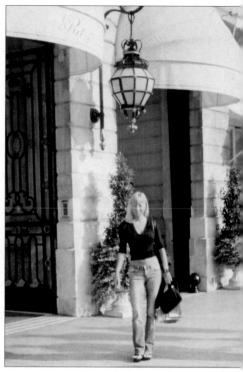

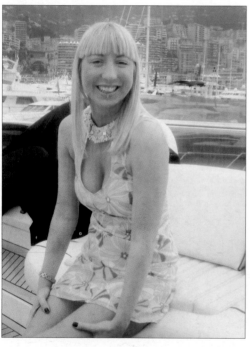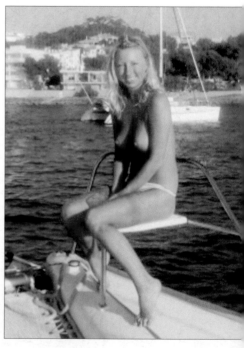

Above left: Another escort date abroad, this time in Hong Kong.

Above right: I was lucky enough to spend a night for work at the Ritz in Paris. Here I am outside.

Below left: Monaco race time in 2007.

Below right: On a client's boat in Majorca.

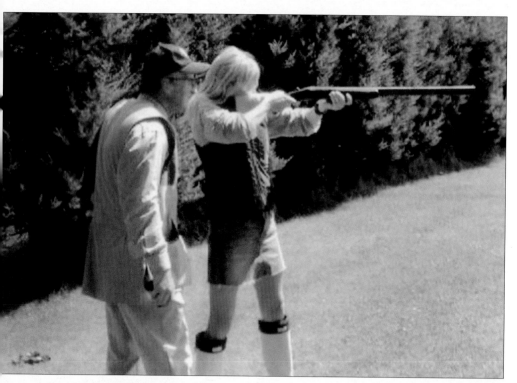

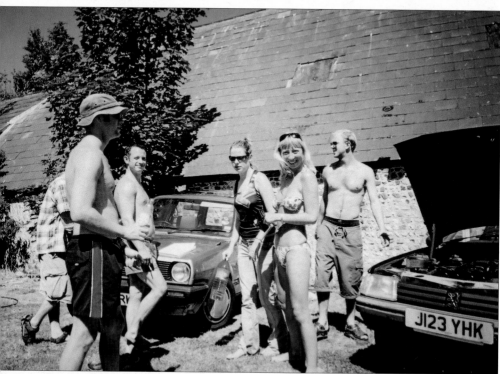

Above: Clay pigeon shooting at the beautiful Thornbury Castle.

Below: The farm gang back together again! Here's some of us preparing for a leaving party before my cousin and brother's trip to New Zealand in 2004. I think around 200 people came to that party!

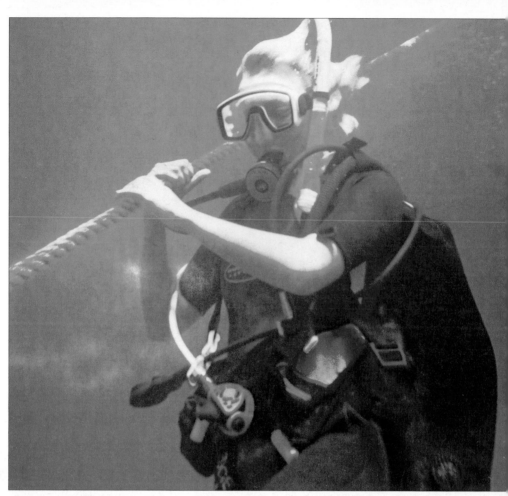

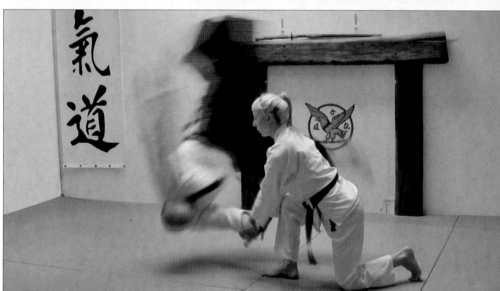

Above: Starting a scuba dive in Egypt.

Below: Throwing my Sensei Kokyunage in Aikido.

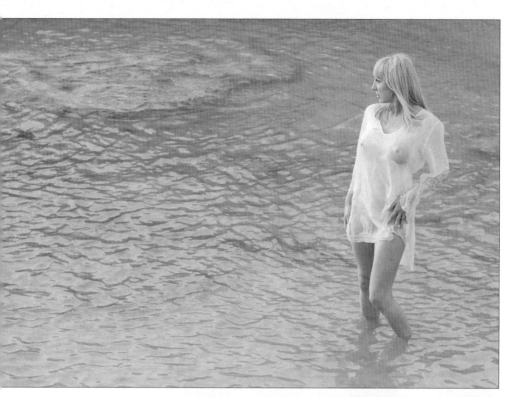

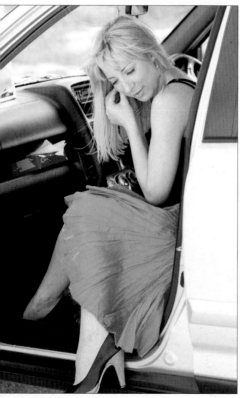

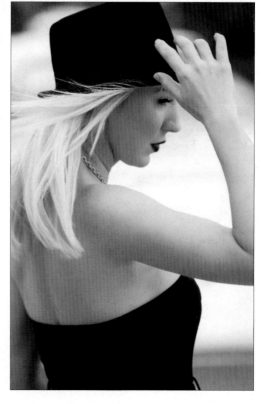

Above and below left: Work photoshoot in Paphos, Cyprus.   © *Andreas (www.evzonas.com)*

Below right: Another work shot, courtesy of Gary Tapp.

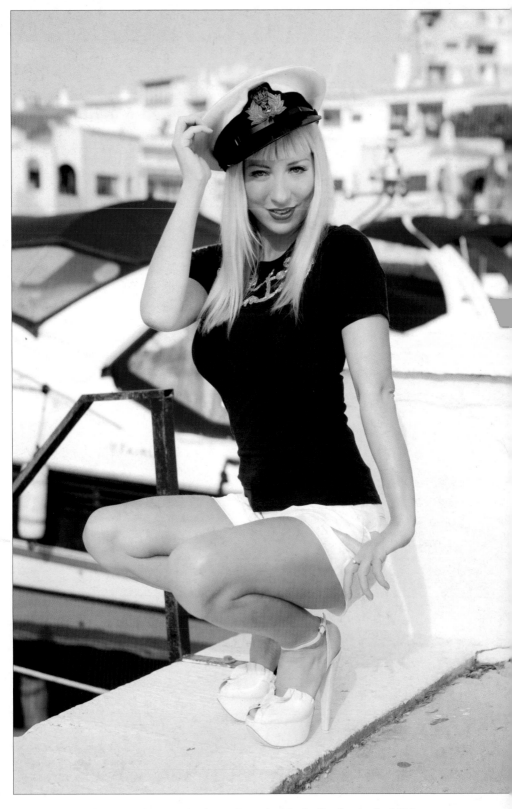

Ahoy there sailor! My last work photoshoot in Marbella, Spain, in 2009.

explained that just as he was ready to meet me, he realised he hadn't been to the bank and didn't have any money. So, he dashed downstairs and the hotel's machine told him he'd already had his daily limit, which meant he had to take his car and find somewhere he could get some more. It certainly gave him something to talk about when I arrived and I'm sure talking about this bit of drama helped him relax.

He then said he had to call his wife. As usual, my heart sank and I thought a bit less of him; he said he'd never booked an escort before and I did believe him. At this point, he didn't offer me the money, but it didn't matter – I'm not too strict with being paid ten minutes into the appointment, unless I think I might not get paid at all. Usually, I wait until I've been to freshen up, which is what I did.

We chatted for about 45 minutes about his work, his house... come to think of it, he never asked about me; I think on this occasion it was nerves. Eventually I got my candles out and asked if we could get the business bit out of the way. I asked him about my website and he said he'd found it very helpful and loved my photos. He asked if I minded his tattoos, and I said I didn't. He apologised, and said he should have checked with me if I was OK with it. It was very sweet of him to mention them, but I told him they were fine.

He kept thanking me for visiting him and saying how beautiful I was. If only I could find a boyfriend who appreciated my beauty and complimented me! We kissed and he was gentle – perfect – and as I teased my tongue lightly in his mouth, he commented that I had a wicked tongue. I've never been told that before – I liked it. I looked into his eyes and gave him a naughty look, gently biting my lower lip, and then I pulled him towards the bed to lie down. Eye contact is very important, not just for conversation, but for intimate moments.

It's no good me trying to avoid eye contact so that I can imagine I'm with Brad Pitt. For guys, part of the fantasy is the idea that you want them and are hungry for them. It's a massive turn-on for them to feel that a stunning woman is hungry for their body.

On the bed it transpired he was a 'bum man – a legs and bum man,' as he said. He unzipped my skirt and I slipped it off. 'Wow,' he kept saying, 'wow!' I'd been slowly teasing the buttons on his shirt undone. This can be quite fiddly if you're trying to kiss someone at the same time and be all sensual! He took off his shirt and trousers too, so I pulled off my top. He lay beside me and admired my belly button ring, before gently turning me on my front so he could nibble my neck and stroke my back; it felt gorgeous.

He stroked my back and over my bum, and unhooked my bra. I straddled him and felt his erection through my panties. I leaned forward to kiss him and my hair fell over his face. He gently sucked each of my nipples and I licked up his neck, nibbled his ears, and then ran my tongue down his body to his briefs. I curled my tongue under the rim of the pants, at the top waistband and underneath, making sure I caught a little of his erect penis, before pulling them down and taking them off.

He said he hadn't been with a woman for so long. His wife was ill and he hadn't had sex or even kissed her properly for over a year. Again, he specifically mentioned that he missed the kissing, and for some guys I think they miss this more than the sex. After the initial disappointment of him cheating on his wife, he went back up in my estimation as I realised that he was just missing being close to someone.

I took him in my mouth and sucked the tip of his large penis.

I looked up at him, but he was lost in the moment, so I carried on. I knew he probably wouldn't last long if he hadn't had sex for over a year so after a few minutes I lay next to him and let him remove my panties and lick me. He did this for a few minutes before I went back down on him. After a few minutes, I asked if he'd like me to get a condom. 'I think you'd better,' was the reply, so I reached over to my little bag, pulled one out and slipped it on, sucking it once the condom was on to keep him erect as I lowered myself on top of him. Even though I was on top, he was thrusting and it felt pretty damn good. I tried to move with him, but it was actually better when I didn't, so I let him do all the work. He started shuddering and making all sorts of noises. I buried my face in his neck – I didn't want to look at him for fear of killing the moment by laughing, which I probably would have done if his facial expressions matched the strange noises! It sounded like one hell of an orgasm – I was quite jealous, actually.

I slowly dismounted and left him to sort himself out. Please don't flush the condom, I thought, but he did. What is it with guys? I guess around 99% of the ones I see try to flush condoms down the loo. Don't they know they're not biodegradable? If I remember, I often ask them not to flush. One of the few guys I've seen that didn't took his sperm-filled condom home to fill it with water – he said it was to check it didn't leak. Like I might have pierced it, wanting to get pregnant or give him some horrible disease!

We lay for the next 20 minutes chatting, and he kept thanking me, saying I really didn't know how much it meant to him for me to see him. He was so sweet. Next time he promised me dinner!

CHAPTER 19:

Boyfriend Number Three – Steve

For well over a year, I was single before meeting Steve. I met him through one of my neighbours while out on her birthday. Most people called it a night at about midnight, but I ended up staying out and partying with him and his friend Simon. We had a real laugh, and they both ended up staying at my place.

Steve and I became good friends. He knew what I did for a living, as he'd asked on the night we met; he was always up for going out and I didn't know many people in Nottingham at the time. After we'd seen each other a couple of times, he said that he fancied me. I asked him what he wanted from me and he said he'd like a relationship. Although he was very sweet (tall, skinny, with an attractive, boyish face), initially I didn't fancy him, so I told him that all I could offer would be friendship. We became very close, to the point that we were seeing each other three or four times a week; we even went away together, but nothing happened. Even though I was quite horny on a few occasions, I managed to resist, and I have so much respect for him because he never tried anything. We'd lie together and cuddle, but never went any further.

After a drunken night out, he confessed that he hadn't had sex for a while. By this point he'd really grown on me and I fancied him like mad, so I joked that as he was a mate, I'd help him out. I told him it was a one-off, though, and not to expect it to happen again – but I wasn't expecting to enjoy it so much! He is the best kisser I've ever met, although he doesn't believe it when I tell him, and everything about our time in bed was amazing. Afterwards, I knew most definitely it would be happening again!

It was then that I realised that I couldn't have sex outside work without getting too attached. This wasn't a one-night stand with a random stranger – it was someone with whom I was spending a huge chunk of my time. I wasn't at all in control of how I felt. In my head, I was thinking, it's just sex, but this was someone I genuinely cared about and I couldn't help my emotions. We then had a bizarre on/off relationship. I didn't want to commit to him because alarm bells were ringing, telling me that he wasn't right for me, but at the same time I couldn't keep away from him. I realised that I was telling him he wasn't a boyfriend, while still treating him like one. How confusing that must have been.

Deep down, I long to be loved and to be in a relationship, and to have someone it means something to, when I give myself. I loved spending time with Steve because when things were good, they were really good, but eventually I didn't feel things would work out – he never complimented me, and there were other things about him including his 'man moods' that I found difficult to deal with. I care for him very much, but he lacks drive and enthusiasm about life and he sometimes tries to make people feel guilty and sorry for him, so he can sometimes end up wallowing in self-pity and negativity.

When we were going out, I suspect a small part of him liked the fact that his friends assumed I was messing him around and felt sorry for him, but we were both to blame for the lack of success in our 'relationship'. Eventually we had to call it a day – I knew it wouldn't work, and neither of us was moving on because of it. We didn't see each other for about eight months, and now we are just friends, but I don't see or speak to him very often. I care about him very much. He's very good to me and the times I do see him he still helps me out if I need his help and he is able.

Steve wasn't comfortable with my job. He never said much, but I just knew he wasn't. He wouldn't ask me about it, but then he never really asked me about anything. Instead, he would ask me how long I planned to escort, but I couldn't tell him because I didn't (and still don't) know what I want to do. When I moaned about work, or anything else, he was always there to listen and he loved to comfort me when I was upset.

I think part of him enjoyed seeing me upset because he felt needed. For example, it was Steve that I called when my 'friend' Nas spoke to me like I was a hooker. I got home in tears and he came round straightaway. He was very supportive, but in the long run he did resent giving me that support. Often, he was round at my flat when I'd be going out to work. Looking back, him being there while I was getting ready did make things awkward. I couldn't get in the right frame of mind for work and I would rush around, worrying I'd be late, because I'd want to stay and be with him until the very last minute. Then he'd get annoyed because I was stressed and he would be in a mood if I didn't drop him at his doorstep, even though he was only ten minutes' walk from mine.

He always thought our relationship wasn't balanced; that he did so much for me, while I did nothing for him. I'd ask him to help me with things because I knew part of him liked me to need his help, but then he'd say he was putting more into the relationship than me. The sad thing was, he didn't acknowledge that I cooked for him, gave him lifts, made him feel good about himself, made him laugh, and was a genuine friend and lover; he'd just focus on the negatives.

If I ever complimented him, he'd think I was lying, just trying to get him to compliment me. Yes, I did want him to compliment me, but I was being myself. I like to make people feel good - hence why I'm good at my job. I don't lie, so any compliment I give is genuine, but he was so insecure he didn't believe me.

Maybe he didn't feel he was good enough for me and was worried I would find someone else, but all this negative behaviour just pushed me away. Some of his 'friends' thought this, as they assumed I was with him for some ulterior motive, which in retrospect is an insult to him as it's suggesting they thought he wasn't good enough for me, so they fuelled his lack of confidence. As I said, the more I got to know him, the more I fancied him – I don't think men understand this. As the months ticked by, I went from initially not being attracted to him at all to fancying the pants off him. I thought he had a lovely face, but I'm convinced he didn't believe me when I told him so. Drunk, he'd be a different person: kind, loving, affectionate – even complimentary. I used to enjoy picking him up from the pub, because he'd be a bit tipsy and I'd be sober. His barriers were down because of the drink and he'd say nice things and be very complimentary. I'd tell him to repeat it all in the morning, if he meant it. He never did. Come the morning his barriers were back in place. Most women hate seeing their partners drunk, but I didn't mind it. If only he could have been the same way sober. If he had, I believe we could have had a successful relationship.

Even when we weren't officially 'boyfriend and girlfriend', we'd always sleep together and people thought of us as a couple. I went to various weddings with him and I think he found it very difficult to deal with the fact I was so honest about my job. He never said anything, but I suspect he found it embarrassing because of people's judgemental reactions. I really wouldn't have a problem going out with a male escort, but I think it must dent a guy's pride a bit, going out with the female version. When we had sex, I know he'd wonder if I was the same as at work. Of course I wasn't! You can't compare the two. Having sex with a boyfriend is completely different because emotions and feelings are involved. He never asked me outright, though and I didn't bring the subject up because I wasn't sure he'd understand if I tried to explain.

The common denominator with all my long-term boyfriends is one way or another, they've had troubled childhoods and I suspect this is one of the reasons why things haven't worked out. I haven't gone out on the hunt for a man who doesn't have a good relationship with his family – it's just turned out that way. In future, I think I'd better check out the family situation early on! Also, none of them owned their own property when we were together, so I suppose that says something; the fact that they don't want any responsibilities shows a lack of commitment and maturity.

I've been single now for over three years and I'm happier than I've ever been. I'm sure when the time is right, Mr Right will find me. What I really want is to be wooed! I know this sounds old-fashioned, but I want someone to really want me, to do whatever it takes to get me and to sweep me off my feet. For the right person, I know I have a lot to offer. Being independent, I need someone who isn't threatened by this, someone who isn't afraid to compliment me, support me and push me to get the best for myself. I'd offer the same and more in return. Although I'm independent, I still like to feel protected and looked after. I do want to have kids and I'm aware of my biological clock ticking, but I'm not going to force the situation. At the moment, I'm concentrating on this book and ending the escorting chapter of my life, before I can even think about settling down and having kids. If I haven't found my Mr Right in the next few years, I might have to have a rethink – I've got a few male friends who I'm sure would help me out!

Diary: September 2008

I dashed out of the apartment in London Bridge to meet my date for the evening. It wasn't our first date, so I didn't mind meeting him at the restaurant. I had booked us in at Roast for a five-hour dinner date and was bang on time at 5 o'clock, but there was no sign of him. I was disappointed because I always think if someone's a gentleman, they try to make sure they're there before you, and he hadn't contacted me to tell me he might be late.

As I sat down, I caught the barman's eye and he came over, gave me a flirty smile and left the drinks menu. I was in London 'on tour'. I had booked an apartment and had three dinner dates arranged. These work in the same way as my usual dates, except my clients come back with me to the apartment rather than me visiting them at a hotel. I'd booked a 4-star apartment as I was there for a few days, and it would be much nicer than being stuck in a poky hotel room. At the apartment I had washing and cooking facilities, a lounge, a dining area and even a DVD player and Sky TV. I was lucky enough to have a balcony, too – it's often cheaper to book a decent apartment than a good hotel.

A work friend of mine was in London, too so we both had some social time together and were able to chat between clients and have a whinge and gossip. Norman, my date, is extremely hard work and emotionally draining. Not only does he suffer from severe SMS, he also mumbles! I can't hear a word he says, and when you're surrounded by noisy people in a public place, it's quite frustrating; it means I have to concentrate really hard to try and lip-read for a good three or four hours. It's exhausting!

Anyhow, my waiter had been eyeing me at the bar, and as soon as I put the menu down and looked up he was over like a shot. I couldn't decide which of the two cocktails I wanted, so I asked his advice and he recommended the Berry Blitz. When he brought it over, he waited for my approval before launching into a conversation about who I was waiting for and whether I'd eaten there before. He was flirting, and I wondered what the tall, dark, handsome young man would think when my date arrived: geeky, sweaty, mumbling Norman! I still hadn't heard from him and now, it was nearly ten past.

As my phone started ringing, I grabbed it, thinking it must be Norman. 'Wanker' was calling me. I clicked to voicemail, but he didn't leave a message. If you look at an escort's phone, we have all sorts of names for callers we want to avoid. I actually have one called 'Avoid', then there's 'Persistent' and 'Idiot'. Usually, I get confused as to which name belongs to which person, but it doesn't matter. They're all calls to be avoided, and if these guys leave messages, I won't reply to them. They're usually people I haven't met, who have left me dodgy messages, or someone I've briefly spoken to and had problems with, so I know I won't agree to see them.

'Wanker' is a guy who contacted me recently about a platonic date (one where there's no private time at all), and I spoke to him but put the phone down when he started making very specific requests, saying he wanted me to take my shoe off and massage his penis with my toes while we were in a restaurant. He then repeatedly texted me to apologise, saying he'd really like to see me. So, his number got saved as 'Wanker'.

The waiter bought over the food menu and gave his recommendations before going back to the bar to serve. I finished my drink, and ordered a champagne cocktail. I still hadn't heard from Norman. I wasn't about to chase him – after all, he was paying for the time. I wasn't about to let him stay any later, though, especially as he hadn't even had the courtesy to call. He worked round the corner so I knew he wasn't stuck on the Underground with no reception.

Norman finally arrived, sweating as I'd predicted, but also smelling strongly of B.O. He plonked himself down next to me – by this time it was half past five. Believe it or not, he was late because he'd been showering! He absolutely stank, so I can't imagine he used any soap and he definitely doesn't use deodorant or cologne. He'd been held up at work and had booked into the same block as me to stay over; he hadn't thought to let me know. Selfish SMS, say no more!

By 6.05p.m., he was agitated and hungry, so we moved to our table, only to be told we'd have to vacate it by 8p.m., which I thought was extremely rude, especially as it wasn't mentioned when I'd booked. There was no way I was spending two hours in the apartment with him! I've never made him come and it ends up with him wanking himself off as I can't even get him hard. It's exhausting and unproductive, so I let him do most of the work. If he can't even make himself come, what hope have I got?

He talked about his work, his allergy to plasters, his Games Workshop battles, and every time I tried to talk about me, he stared around the room, making it clear he wasn't interested in what I had to say. He's probably over shadowed at work by strong characters, hence his need to just talk about himself and his total lack of interest in me. I kept asking him to speak up, telling him I couldn't hear him, but he never did. Had he been interested in me, I would have been interested in him, but I was bored stiff listening to him talk – well, mumble – about himself for hours.

By the time we ordered dessert it was past 8p.m., but thankfully we weren't asked to leave the table. He ordered some sort of chocolate dessert and he got it all round his mouth. It was repulsive! I looked and noticed his napkin hadn't been used at all. The first time I met him, by the end of the meal he'd managed to layer up all his courses on his large, full lips: soup, something tomatoey, and cream from an Irish coffee. It was absolutely revolting! This time, I left it a couple of minutes, amusing myself by wondering if he'd notice. He didn't. So, I told him he had chocolate all round his face and said, 'No wonder, you haven't even used your napkin!' Vile table manners are usually standard with SMS men.

By the time we got back to the apartments, we had about an hour. He went to his apartment to collect my envelope and brush his teeth. I'd asked him to brush his teeth after we had our first lunch to get the gunk from his lips, but I still tasted the cream around his mouth when I kissed him... yuck! Back in the bedroom, I put on some music. His armpits stank and I contemplated asking him to shower, but for some reason I didn't. I decided to be assertive and asked if he'd like to give me oral sex, so he did. It felt really good, and I let him do it for about 15 minutes before giving him oral. He never gets an erection and it's really disheartening, so I usually get him to sort himself out. He started wanking as I deep French-kissed him and rubbed my breasts in his face and down his torso. It took 25 minutes of sweating and straining, with his face bright red, before he managed to bring himself off.

I think he thought he'd stay late, so I got up and put on my pyjamas, making it clear I was going to be off to bed. He left about ten past ten, and I opened the window to disperse the lingering sweaty smell and enjoyed a long bath.

CHAPTER 20:

Bad Hygiene
and Inappropriate
Behaviour

My pet hate is bad hygiene. I spend a lot of time preparing for my dates and I'm always fresh, sweet-smelling, shaved and in tip-top condition, so when someone hasn't made the same effort, I just think it's damn rude. I have no respect for guys like that, because they clearly have no respect for me; I think guys should shower before they meet me. And if they feel sweaty during our date, they should shower again before we get intimate.

Please make sure you've eaten, because this is going to get gross... I'm amazed there are grown men who don't know how to wash their bits. Don't they realise they need to pull the foreskin right back and give it a good old clean with lots of soap? I always think circumcised is so much nicer. One guy's bits smelt so bad, I didn't go anywhere near – I wasn't going to ask him to wash it properly, so I just avoided it. The first time we met was for an extended overnight in Bristol. After kissing him and smelling a bit of B.O., I excused myself and went to the bathroom to do my hygiene checks... only to discover the bottom of the shower was dry, the soap was unopened, and the towels hadn't been moved or used. He hadn't even washed! I tried to be subtle and asked if he wanted to shower, but he said he was OK. Talk about not getting the hint! 'So, when *did* you have one?' I inquired. 'This morning,' came the answer. I had met him at 3p.m., and we'd been out for a late lunch; it was now nearer 6p.m. and he stank! So, I had to ask him to have a shower if he wanted things to go any further in the bedroom. Reluctantly, he went in.

We went away numerous times, and once we went to Rome. He'd started showering twice a day, which sorted out the B.O., but I still didn't have sex with him or give him oral or touch him down below because he wasn't washing properly. So, we just cuddled and kissed. Silly man, he didn't know what he was missing!

On our last date in Rome I jumped in the shower, and asked if there was a towel. He gave me a used one – it looked like it had make-up on it, so he said it must be mine. I have no idea why, but I decided to give the towel a quick sniff. It was actually poo! I was fuming. How could anyone do that? I don't get it. Yuck!

I hit the roof. I told him it certainly wasn't my towel, as I wiped and washed myself properly! He stood there, bemused, looking a little embarrassed, but he didn't apologise. I couldn't believe it. Thankfully I never saw him again.

Some guys actually try to trick me, saying they have just showered. They think I'll take their word for it! I then point out that the shower is bone-dry and send them in, telling them to make sure they take their time. Once, I arrived at a date and the guy (single again, have you noticed a trend?) had been out the night before with friends. I'd arrived the following day, about 2p.m., and he hadn't been out of the room all day. The place stank, and I suspected he was wearing the same clothes as the night before, too.

We went out to watch a matinee at the theatre and when he put his arm around me, I could smell his pits – it made me feel sick. When we got back to the hotel, we had an hour or so before dinner. After watching TV for a short while, I told him I couldn't bear it any longer, that he smelt and needed to get in the shower because it was making me feel queasy. He said he'd had a shower, but I didn't believe him. Then he tried to convince me he wasn't a shower-dodger, which he clearly was. There's no excuse for a lack of basic hygiene. It's no wonder he lived on his own and was single. He asked if I knew a good deodorant – I told him he'd have to start with a good soap first!

One guy was in a rush when I arrived for our dinner date and didn't want to 'waste' any time in the shower – so he started washing his pits in the sink! I knew I'd make him shower properly when we came back to the room after dinner, but you can have a quick shower and wash in just a few minutes if need be, so I've no idea why he didn't. He didn't wash properly so we didn't do anything in the bedroom either.

There was also another guy with poor hygiene, someone I saw when I first started escorting. John worked in computing and lived with a bunch of students. He would turn up for our dates casual, with no overnight bag; he didn't even have a toothbrush. I'd say to him that if he didn't bring his toothbrush, then I wouldn't kiss him in the morning. On one occasion he said he was off to the bathroom to brush his teeth, so I listened at the door, but all I could hear was running water. When he came out, I said he obviously hadn't done it and he argued, so I asked to see his toothbrush and of course he didn't have one!

It's like teaching small children. Maybe some guys get a kick out of getting me into 'mother' mode. 'Don't forget to wash behind your ears' and all that. Why do they assume that I'm incredibly stupid? Or is it them? Either way, it tickles me. At the end of the day, it's their loss – I don't mind not kissing, or not giving them sex.

The same guy once asked me to stay with him in his student house because he'd told his flatmates that I was his girlfriend. What a silly thing to do! What if I was out on another date and saw his friends? They'd think I was cheating on him or something, and cause a scene. Fortunately, I didn't bump into any of his housemates when I stayed, but I was pissed off to find he hadn't even tidied up. It was a typical student room, with dirty cups everywhere and half-eaten pizza on the floor. He was paying me £700 for an overnight, yet he lived in an absolute dive. Afterwards, I told him we'd have to go back to staying in hotels because his place was dirty and messy – I just thought it was rude and disrespectful of him to invite me to his home and not even try to make it nice. Fresh sheets and a quick tidy would have been enough.

It's not just bad hygiene that puts me off – some guys' behaviour leaves a lot to be desired. I'm good in most social situations, so I don't mind going out in public on dates, but I like to make sure I'm prepared. As with John, people need to be aware that I may be seen with other people in the future, so I'd always advise them to say I'm a friend rather than a girlfriend.

I once met a guy for an overnight date at his home near London. When he collected me from the station, he asked if I wanted to go to his flying club (I think he wanted to show me off to people he knew, and impress me with his plane). I was a bit dubious and asked if there would be many people there – I was really dressed up as he'd said we'd be going to an upmarket French restaurant, but he was wearing jeans, so I assumed the club was quite casual and he'd be changing for dinner when we went back to his place. At the flying club he showed me his plane and then we sat outside and got a drink from the bar. We were then joined by a couple he knew, and then came all the usual questions. I was totally unprepared and felt extremely uncomfortable, especially as I looked so out of place in what I was wearing. Then, without consulting me, he invited them to join us for dinner!

I couldn't believe it! He decided we'd go straight to a local chain pub instead of the lovely restaurant he'd booked us into – he wasn't going to go back to his place to wash or change, either. The food was disgusting and the social side a disaster. The couple must have been suspicious about him trying to pass me off as his girlfriend – I'd obviously never been mentioned to them and clearly, I knew nothing about him. Once we left the restaurant, I was fuming and let him have a real earful when we got to his car. He apologised, but didn't understand why I was so angry. The rest of the date was fine once we were on our own, but I couldn't believe he'd put me in such an awkward situation.

I used to ask guys what they wanted me to wear, but I found that people would be far too specific, or they'd ask me to wear something smart and then turn up wearing jeans. So, now I usually ask what they're planning to wear and I find out what kind of place we'll be going to, just so I can be sure to dress appropriately. I remember once meeting Jack, my accountant regular. I breezed into this posh hotel in Birmingham, dressed up and looking glam. There were a number of businessmen in the lobby; I knew some were watching me, looking to see who I was meeting. I strode up to the bar and Jack was there, in a T-shirt that was far too small (his huge, veiny belly was sticking out) and cargo trousers! He stood up to greet me, and I noticed his spotty bum cleavage and wished I could have seen the businessmen's faces!

I asked if he was changing for dinner and he said no. So, I said it would have been nice if he'd told me he wouldn't be dressing up and then I could have done the same. When we met before, he'd always dressed smartly. There's no way we'll ever look like a couple, but at least if we're wearing similar clothing we hopefully look like acquaintances or work colleagues.

When we ate out, he repeatedly ate with his mouth open and talked with his mouth full. I tried to be patient and subtle by looking at his mouth with the food churning around, instead of his eyes, when he was speaking. He didn't get the hint, so I tried shaking my head disapprovingly while looking at his mouth as food spluttered out; it was really making me feel sick. He still didn't get the hint and carried on speaking, so I blatantly had to ask him not to speak with a mouthful of food and told him I didn't want to see the contents of his mouth. I have never met such a disgusting eater! I even stopped trying to make conversation while we ate because I didn't want to encourage him to talk. Have these guys not heard the old saying, 'manners maketh the man?' Well, it's absolutely true.

Another guy, an ex-regular from Liverpool, used to have really poor table manners. I'd see him once a month for a couple of nights at his house, and I had to tell him not to speak with his mouth full, too. Often I got food flying into my face, or onto my plate, from his mouth. He spent so much money booking me, but his towels and dressing gowns were threadbare, and his kitchen wasn't clean. He'd give me cups and cutlery that hadn't even been washed properly. Really, he should have got himself a cleaner with the money he spent on escorts!

We'd go to the theatre and do all sorts of things, but when we were back at his house, there was nothing to do. He wouldn't put the TV on, so I'd be bored and either read the paper, have a bath or go to bed for a snooze. He was so emotionally draining, because he wanted me to be 100% focused on him all the time. In the end, I just ran out of conversation. One day, when we were at his local supermarket, it tickled me when someone asked if I was his daughter!

A couple of years ago, he contacted me again and I said I'd see him if he booked a hotel. He asked why, and I tried to be tactful, saying I'd be more comfortable if we stayed there but he didn't get it, so I ended up saying his threadbare towels and dirty kitchen weren't really appealing. He didn't want to meet up again, which was fine, but he must have understood what I was telling him because I heard that another escort went to visit him and his place was spotless, with fluffy new towels!

One of the worst bookings I had was when I went to see someone I hadn't met before, Charles, who had inquired about me visiting him at home. He couldn't verify his address, but he pointed me to his company website, where there was lots of interesting information about him, along with a photograph. He was a top financial adviser and looked like he was in his fifties or sixties. In the build-up to our date I was convinced he was the kind of person I usually enjoy meeting. He seemed to care about my comfort, he said he wanted me to wear whatever I felt comfortable in (a good sign), and he had booked a restaurant, but said I could change it if there was something I preferred, so I had built up an image of a kind, thoughtful, well-to-do older guy.

We exchanged a few texts, and when I told him what time I thought I'd get to his apartment, he said he might still be in the bath. Forty-five minutes before I was due to arrive, he messaged me and said he was just getting into the bath. This rang alarm bells; did he think we would jump straight into bed for a session before dinner? Why would it take him over 45 minutes to bathe? I arrived bang on time into London, but just in case he was still getting ready, I waited at the station for 15 minutes. I called him and he said he was ready, so I jumped in a cab. As soon as we entered his apartment, he said, 'I know you don't like slobbery kisses, but...' and proceeded to try and give me a slobbery kiss. Yuck!

I thought he was an idiot from that moment. Why would you do something to someone that you know they really don't like? I pulled away, wiped his slobber on the back of my hand, and he asked what I wanted to do. I said I'd like to go for a drink before dinner, so he quickly showed me around his pad and then we went out to a bar. He was a really interesting guy, and also seemed very interested in me. The restaurant was a gorgeous French place, but half-empty, and I suspected that he had arranged the meal for 8.30p.m. so that we could have a sex session before dinner. I never do that, even with regulars, and before I even confirm a date I always make it clear that I like to dine first.

The meal was delicious. He ordered wine and champagne, which I thought was a bit much. I knew I'd need to keep my eye on my glass because the waiters just keep topping them up when you're not looking! During the meal he said that I looked like someone who spoke my mind, and wouldn't do anything I didn't want to do. I agreed, and he seemed to understand and respect the person that I am. Then we went back to his apartment. He never offered me a drink – I would have only had water, anyway, but it's always nice to be asked. I lit candles and put them around his room, and he put some music on. We started kissing, and straightaway, he took all my clothes off. I don't like that – I like to take my time, and he was too eager. He was getting a little too close for comfort without a condom on, but he said it was OK and he wasn't trying to put it in. I said it was a good job, as I would be straight out of there if he did!

He groped me for a few minutes and then asked if I had a condom. I just thought he was a total prick – I couldn't understand how someone could switch from being a thoughtful, caring person to a selfish idiot. I decided I would give him a bit of oral sex before I put the condom on, but he told me to just do what he'd asked! If I'd been closer to home I would have left, but I didn't want to wander round London so late at night, so I decided to put up with it. I put on the condom, and hoped he would come quickly so I could get off to bed. Already I'd decided I was having the spare room! So, I tried my best to maintain eye contact with him, and tell him how good it felt with him inside me. That did the trick, and he came after a few minutes.

Afterwards, he tried to give me oral and asked if I'd come, and I said probably not now as it was late. He told me not to worry, that we would try again later. I pointed out that as it was nearly 1a.m. I'd be going to bed in a few minutes, and told him that an overnight date didn't mean sex all night! He said he had certain expectations, but I told him the more he put into a meeting of this kind, the more he would get out of it. I then said I was sleeping in the spare room and that I'd go in and give him a cuddle in the morning.

He looked pissed off, but as far as I was concerned, why should it matter where I sleep? He had annoyed me so much and I knew he'd be pestering me for more sex at some point during the night. The bed was small and I couldn't bear to be anywhere near him because of how he had treated me. I went to the spare room, taking my suitcase with me, because I'm sure he would have gone through it to try and take his money back. I left it directly behind the door so I would wake up, if he tried to come in.

At 7.15a.m. he came rapping on my door, saying, 'Time to get up!' like I was in the Army! I couldn't believe it. Irritated and disorientated, I was feeling more than a little worse for wear. I snapped that I was having another hour. About 15 minutes later, he did the same thing again and told me I had to get out because he had a train to catch. I knew he was lying to get me out. I didn't even have time to shower – my eyes were half-closed, my hair all over the place. I couldn't believe what he was doing. How rude! He didn't even check if I'd be able to get home. There I was, out on the Strand with my suitcase, still half-asleep at 7.45a.m.

If he genuinely had to catch a train that early (which I know he didn't), he should have told me at the time of booking because in that case I wouldn't have visited him at home. I would have asked him to arrange a hotel so that I could stay longer. He was just annoyed that he didn't get his own way the night before; that he didn't have me up like a sex machine all night. I'm so glad I stayed in the spare room and I was more than happy to get away from him!

I always used to find it awkward, asking for the money on bookings. I'd never ask for it, and never count it either. I know I shouldn't have felt bad about it, but I did. It took me a couple of bad experiences before I finally started asking for the money at the beginning of the date and counting it out in front of the gentleman. That way, if it's short, I can't be accused of hiding it. Sometimes a date will accidentally give me too much, so it doesn't always work out to my benefit.

The first time I was swindled out of money, it was to the tune of £700, which at that time was the amount I charged for an overnight date. I was approached by a gentleman who claimed to work for the government: he said he was looking to meet someone on a regular basis; who would be put on a payroll. I would need to be exclusively available and able to travel at short notice. Intrigued and excited, I decided to meet him for a coffee to discuss matters further.

We met in Derby at a pub close to the station. He was about 50, grey, and balding, and wearing a smart grey suit; he showed me official documents and his passport, which proved his identity. We spent about an hour chatting, and I told him that before we could take things to the next level it would be advisable to book me for an overnight, to check that we could get along over a longer period. I explained this would need to be a paid booking. We arranged an overnight date at Gatwick Airport and it took me hours to get to him as the trains were delayed. He didn't offer me the money upfront, and I didn't ask for it. We went out for dinner and then retired to the room. In the morning, he said he hadn't slept, which I believed as on the odd occasion when I'd woken in the night, he was bolt upright in bed! I wondered whether he was on drugs.

We had more fun in the morning, and when I was due to leave I asked him for my money. I was fuming when he said he didn't have it and would pay it into my bank account. There was nothing I could do – it was my fault for not asking for it earlier. Needless to say, the money never arrived and eventually I gave up ringing and asking him for it.

That story has an interesting twist, though. A few years later, a gentleman friend from one of the review sites booked me for the evening, for a trip to London. We stayed in one of my favourite hotels there, the Sanderson. That evening we were going out with another gentleman and his date, an escort (who I had met a few times), her female friend, and a gentleman who had her on a payroll and was buying her lavish gifts. She had spoken about him on numerous occasions – he had paid off the mortgage on her house, and had bought her a brand new sports car, diamonds and much more; she travelled with him all over the world, and also took her friend. Both got paid for their time.

We turned up at Attica in London to meet up with everyone, and there was a real party spirit, with numerous bottles of pink champagne on ice. I was introduced to everyone there – including Andrew, the guy who'd ripped me off several years earlier. 'It's nice to meet you, Andrew,' I said, with a knowing smile. To say I was shocked was an understatement. I told my date about him, and he said to let him stew for a bit. I left it for hours without saying anything to him – I wanted to choose my timing very carefully. I'm sure he knew that Carol would have been really angry, if she knew he'd ripped me off. She was a feisty character, and it would have reflected really badly on him to have been so tight with me, seeing as he clearly had plenty of money! So I kept quiet and let him wonder whether I'd said anything to her. He kept plying us all with champagne – maybe he was hoping to get me so drunk, I would forget the whole thing.

Soon I found myself standing next to him, away from the

THE GIRLFRIEND EXPERIENCE

rest of our crowd. 'So,' I said. 'Andrew, how are you?' He shifted about a bit, and looked extremely uncomfortable. I loved watching him squirm. 'Very well, thanks, and you?' he asked innocently. 'We have a bit of unfinished business,' I said. He agreed, and glanced around to check that no one was looking. 'Well, that £700 has gained a bit of interest; it's now £1,000,' I informed him. He quickly gave me his number, asked me to call him the next day, and promised it would all be sorted out. Within a couple of days, I had the money. It was worth waiting years just to see the look on his face when he was introduced to me! And of course the £300 interest was handy, although I kicked myself for not asking for more. I think he would have paid me anything I'd asked, just to keep his little indiscretion quiet.

I'm a firm believer in what goes around, comes around, and he certainly got his comeuppance. Less than a year after I got my money back, he was rumbled by the government. His face was plastered over the papers, along with the story of how he had squandered Government money on high-class escorts. He had ripped the government off to the tune of hundreds of thousands of pounds, and found himself in jail.

Previously, I've been offered the chance to win a car by someone who claimed that he could choose the winners in prize draw competitions; he then said he wanted me to pay for the car in dates. Unbelievable! That was while I was still known as 'Barbie', so no doubt he thought I'd be a dizzy blonde. I told him, 'When I have the car, I'll see you.' He actually expected me to take his word for it, and to start seeing him for nothing! Once, I was even asked if I would accept high street gift vouchers as payment!

It's usually rich people who push for discounts and try and get freebies. Guys with average earnings are usually more respectful and don't ask. Some want a discount if they're looking for a holiday companion. They think if they're paying for first-class travel and a luxury 5-star, then they shouldn't have to pay much for a lady, because it's 'a holiday'. It might be a vacation for them, but if they expect me to be there all the time, and be intimate with them at some point, it's work for me, and if they expect me to work, then it's not a 'free holiday'!

I love kissing. I think kissing should be slow and inquisitive, and when it's right, I can kiss for hours. Great kissers vary their technique and read signals from the other person. So, if their partner is easing away, they don't keep following them and forcing them to keep kissing, they let them move away. It might be a short, teasing pause, or perhaps their partner wants to kiss elsewhere. I love nibbling necks and ears – and having mine nibbled, too. Gently probing tongues are nice, and also gentle sucking of the upper and lower lips. However, I find it amazing that so many guys can't kiss. I absolutely hate forceful, slobbery kissing. Having my head clamped by someone's arm into a kiss is not pleasant, but I'm really surprised how many men do this. Every boyfriend I've had has been an amazing kisser and has never been forceful with kissing, because for me, it's such a turn-off.

In my work I've had odd kissers who almost kiss like a fish. They make their lips firm and just open and close them against mine, but the most common bad kissing trait is slobber. Often I have to wipe the saliva off my face, and I make a point of doing this obviously in the hope they will stop slobbering. I would say that unfortunately 90% of the guys I kiss are awful, slobbery kissers. It's no wonder their wives don't want to kiss them or have sex! If they could sort their kissing out, they might find they actually turn their wives on, but most of the time it's such a turn-off and I dislike it immensely. I would rather give oral sex than kiss them on the lips; I can understand why so many ladies in this profession don't kiss.

The lady I sometimes go to for facials had a date with a guy recently, and his kissing was slobbery and disgusting, but she never said anything to him at the time – she's just been avoiding his phone calls ever since! I told her she should tell him, because if no one does, he probably won't ever have any success with women and he will be confused as to why.

Apart from bad kissing, the worst thing in the bedroom is when guys think they can move me round like a rag doll. I get very stroppy if someone just wants to move me around and orchestrate me. I've literally had people turn me over and put my body into certain positions, like I'm an object. I also find 'dirty' talk when I'm working hilarious. It's just *so* cheesy! I had one guy who wanted me to tell him his cock was really big, and I just laughed and asked him why – because it wasn't! Dirty talk really isn't my bag and I find it hard to keep a straight face. 'Ooooh, you love sucking that cock, don't you?' Whatever!

I once had a disaster date that should never have happened. Looking back, alarm bells started ringing when I was asked to paint my nails bright red and bring stockings, suspenders, a pair of glasses and another set of lingerie. You're probably thinking that's no big deal, but after seven years in the business, the word 'control freak' springs to mind. I don't like being told what to do or what to wear, so it puts me on edge straightaway. I could have, and probably should have, said 'no' there and then, but I didn't and so we arranged a date.

I'm used to people saying, 'Wear what you feel comfortable in', not giving me a checklist of things. If a gentleman is so specific, he's likely to think that it's all about him because he's paying, and that's not the kind of person I enjoy spending time with. Throughout our emails he reminded me about the red nails, and also added strappy sandals to the ever-growing list. I joked that I'd need a suitcase and hoped I'd remember everything, because if I didn't, I had a feeling he would send me packing! He said he had a foot-and-leg fetish, so I assumed that meant he would be spending a lot of time appreciating my feet and legs. I didn't think this would be an easy job, but I thought it would be quite different, and assumed there would be lots of leg and foot worship. It wasn't something I had experienced much of before, so I was quite intrigued.

I arrived at the hotel and knocked on his door. He was shorter than me, about 5'4", dressed in a sharp suit, and quite attractive with a confident air. It transpired he was a financier. Over a glass of champagne, we chatted about his work and mine. I had arrived at 7p.m. for a four-hour dinner date; I didn't feel rushed and we took our time over dinner. He respected the way I run my business and was very interested; he also seemed to understand me as a person. I really enjoyed his company, and I almost forgot about all the things I'd had to bring; I was confident we would have a lovely evening.

When we got back to the room, I went to the bathroom to change. I walked out and he sat down and admired my outfit. He stroked me up and down my legs. He smelt lovely, always a good start, and his kissing was soft and felt delicious. I was bending down to kiss him as he was sitting down. I sat opposite him on the sofa and he put my legs in the air and removed my shoes, while sucking my toes. He left big clumps of food on them, which wasn't very pleasant! After dinner, I'd brushed my teeth and he clearly hadn't, as he seemed to be flossing with my nylons! He noticed, and I know he hoped I hadn't, because as he pretended to massage my toes he was actually trying to get the white bits of potato off my stocking!

He pulled my knickers to one side and probed my pussy, then asked me to get his cock out. I did, and he put it to my mouth for me to suck. I was lying down, and he was standing over me. He wanted me to scratch his balls at the same time, quite roughly. After a few minutes, I moved my mouth away and he asked me to suck it again. I had moved away because I wanted to do something else, so I was a bit perturbed. I said I was starting to feel very uncomfortable with the way things were going – I could sense this would not be a two-way meeting, more, 'I'm paying, and this is what I want'. When I stopped again, he just stood there, waiting, his erect cock in my face and his hands behind his back. Well, that was it. I stopped and told him I felt uncomfortable with what was happening.

I tried to think how best to put into words what I wanted to say without being too blunt and making him feel bad; that I wasn't used to meetings like this. I said I felt like he was controlling me, and that I didn't expect to be told what to do.

We spent a good half-hour analysing what had gone wrong and how it could have been avoided. He was used to seeing girls for two hours and having oral sex twice, and was obviously used to them doing as they were told. I told him I was used to the opposite: to meeting someone and it being a two-way pleasure trip, with both parties equally involved, creating a build-up to one amazing orgasm, hopefully for both. I'm old-fashioned, and think it should be ladies first, anyway!

He is a member on one of the review sites and there was nothing in any of my reviews to suggest I was into one-way, PSE meetings. If he'd done his homework properly, he should have known that I wasn't the kind of person that he would enjoy spending time with. This is part of what it says on my site:

If you...
• are disrespectful
• are forceful and pushy
• don't care about my feelings and comfort
• have an obsessive or controlling nature
• are looking for a PSE (Porn Star Experience)

... then I am not the lady for you, and in some instances such behaviour on a date will lead to me terminating the meeting.

In the bedroom he was all of these things! Obviously it was awkward and I wasn't sure what to do. I did think he was a genuinely nice guy, so I didn't want to leave it, with both of us disappointed, so I suggested we start again. I went back to the bathroom and came out again, and we started over, but this time he didn't tell me to do anything. It wasn't long before he came. Under the circumstances, it wouldn't be fair to write a review, so he decided not to. We both learnt something and I don't think either of us will make the same mistake again.

This is a classic example of how escorts differ. I have escort friends who assume their job is to perform sexually, so they would have just got on with the job and not had an issue with it. I don't advertise that I sell sex, and my job is to offer good company, so I insist on being treated with respect.

I also dislike public displays of affection while I'm working. I don't mind linking arms with guys, but if you're holding hands you look like a couple and I do like to be discreet in public. It's for this reason that I try to avoid holding hands. I'm very tactile, so I don't have a problem with being close to people generally; it's just kissing, holding hands or groping in public that I don't like. Anything non-sexual is fine. I'm most affectionate with guys that I'm very comfortable with, those that are relaxed, not full-on. Personally, I think it's rude to try to snog someone the minute they walk through the door.

I'm so old fashioned – I want to get to know someone a bit first. Once, I had an awful dinner date with a guy who immediately tried to kiss and grope me. I pushed him away, but all through dinner he kept trying to put his hand up my skirt, even though a family was sitting next to us. It was awful! Afterwards, we went for a little walk and he tried to do the same. In the end, I had to be very abrupt with him and told him that I didn't like it.

I was on a date in Italy once and the guy constantly touched my fingers and hands while we were eating. It was quite annoying: God help anyone who gets between me and my food! At one point, when he started kissing both my hands and sliding my fingers into his mouth while I had my knife in my hand, I whipped my hands away and asked what he was doing. I felt really uncomfortable as we were surrounded by people eating. As an onlooker, it would have certainly put me off my meal! I suppose he wanted it to look like we were a touchy-feely real couple, but it was a total turn-off!

Guys who constantly want assurance are difficult to be around. When they say things like, 'You really don't want to be here, do you?' it actually makes me feel that way. It's incredibly uncomfortable. Or, 'I bet you don't like being seen with an ugly oldie like me?' They forget that generally women are less shallow when it comes to looks. How often do you see an unattractive lady with an attractive guy? Often, I see unattractive men with stunning women, but rarely the other way round. I really am interested in getting to know the people I meet and visual looks are not important to me. Of course if they're attractive *and* a nice guy, it's always a bonus!

The opposite are those who are intrusive about my private life. I don't mind a few questions, but sometimes it's too much. There's plenty to talk about without either party getting personal. And then there are the guys who feel sorry for me because they think I must have had all sorts of bad experiences. I find it extremely patronising – I'm very choosy about who I see, and although I've written about a few bad experiences here, they are few and far between considering that I've been escorting for eight years.

I've heard stories a million times worse from other ladies. One Northern Angels girl let herself get so battered and bruised from someone having sex with her that she was in agony and couldn't sit down; she had to have over four weeks off work! She decided to tell everyone on the public forum, and although I didn't know her, I immediately called to offer her sympathy and advise her on what to do in a similar situation in the future. This was not something she should have put on a public forum. Hindsight is a wonderful thing though, isn't it? If it was that bad, she should have walked out with the cash! I asked why she didn't use lubrication and she said she didn't think guys liked it. I don't care whether they like it or not, if I need it or want to use it, then I do. It's not like I just use lubrication for work – I always use it to play with boyfriends, too. She said she didn't want a bad review! Sod the reviews – our health, well-being and self-respect are worth far more than a review. I won't compromise on these things for anyone.

Diary: February 2008

'I'm sorry, there's no reservation for a Mr O'Donnelly.' 'Could you please double-check? I have the room number here – it's 1001,' I said. 'Just a minute... No, I'm sorry, there's nothing under that name.' Cursing, I hung up and decided to call the restaurant next door to check the reservation there. We were supposedly booked in for dinner at 8.45p.m. When I was told again that there was no reservation, my heart sank. I was sitting in my car, all dolled up, wearing a fitted grey dress, tight leather jacket and knee boots ready for my dinner date. I cursed myself for not checking earlier. A timewaster... great!

I called him and expected to get his voicemail, but he picked up after a couple of rings, so I challenged him. 'Well, the room's all booked and paid for,' he said, rather jovially, 'and I've made a reservation for dinner.' I didn't know what to say. 'Can you give me a few minutes and I'll call you back?' he asked. I called the hotel again to say that I had spoken to Mr O'Donnelly and he was definitely in room 1001. It turned out he was also on a call to the hotel at the same time. I decided to take a gamble because if I didn't leave there and then, I would be late. Even worse, he might be late, too, and ask me to stay longer. We were due to meet for a dinner date at 8.30p.m. and I didn't want our time to run over. He called me back to say it was all sorted, but that he may be a few minutes late; he'd told the hotel that I might arrive first and said they would give me the key.

I arrived bang on time, parked and teetered in my heels across the road to the hotel. 'I've come to collect a key for room 1001 – my partner has said he called you,' I said to the lady behind the desk. 'Actually,' I added, 'I was told he wasn't staying here when I called.' 'I have the reservation here,' said the lady. 'Why couldn't you find him when I called earlier?' 'Because he hadn't checked in yet,' she answered, as if that explained everything. Surely he would have been in the system? I even had his room number!

The receptionist wanted me to fill in a form with my name, address and other personal details. I could have made up some information, but decided to tell them it would be best if he filled it in. After assuring the receptionist that 'my partner' would be arriving in five minutes, she reluctantly she gave me the key. Knowing the hotel quite well, I made my way to the lifts. I put the TV on in the room and settled into an armchair to wait for my date. By 8.45 I was a little irritated, but only because I was hungry and I still wasn't sure if he would actually turn up. But if he wanted to pay for me to sit in a hotel room and watch TV, this would be easiest job ever! He called to say he was just around the corner and would be arriving in a couple of minutes. By 8.55, he still hadn't arrived, and I got another call saying the same thing – he was just around the corner. By 9p.m.

I was really pissed off and wondering whether this was some sort of joke. What if he didn't arrive and I didn't get paid? I couldn't understand it – I thought it was very odd.

Had I been 100% sure he would arrive and pay me, then I would have been OK, but I started to think he was winding me up, so I called him. 'Where exactly are you?' I asked, looking out on the road to see if I could spot him in the dark. 'I'm on the corner by the hotel,' he said, and apologised. 'You said that last time!' I snapped back. 'I'm really sorry about this, but I am on the corner – I had to stop to take a call. I'll be with you in two minutes,' he replied. 'If you have to park your car, you won't be here in two minutes. I'll see you in ten,' I said, rather huffily, before hanging up.

Sure enough, ten minutes later, I heard the key card in the door. I could hear him struggling, so I opened the door a fraction and then pushed it again as if to close it, saying cheekily, 'Not today, thank you,' before opening it fully. Standing there was a jolly-looking Irishman with a big, round, smiley face and glasses, dressed smartly in a full-length overcoat. He apologised profusely and looked quite flustered. He said that someone had crashed into his car, and he'd gone to the wrong hotel. All sorts of excuses poured out, and I wasn't sure what to believe. It just seemed odd.

He then proceeded to count out my fee in tens! Great! Instead of putting them in piles of hundreds, he counted £300 in one pile. Then he counted out another big pile of tens, making £600 in total. He had wanted an overnight, but as I had an early hair appointment the next day, I had told him that I would meet him, but it would just be a dinner date. If he'd have been free earlier, I'd have suggested a 5-hour date, but at 8.30 I knew I wouldn't be able to stay up until

1.30, so I said I'd see him for four hours. 'You've given me too much,' I said, hoping that for all the messing around, he might tell me not to worry. Thankfully, he did.

I told him that I was starving, so we made our way down to dinner. Linking my arm with his, I grinned at him. He was a nice guy, and I was happy now I'd got paid, so I could settle in to enjoy our date. In the restaurant he started talking about himself and his successful companies (probably another single guy, I thought). Although he looked older, it turned out that he was only 36. I learnt that at the age of 21, he was living in a £1 million pound house. He could run a mile in under six minutes and used to be very athletic; he enjoyed playing and watching rugby, and yes, he was single! This was his first time with an escort, he said.

He wasn't even looking at the menu. I was struggling to stay interested in his conversation and I knew I wouldn't relax until we'd ordered food. When the waitress brought our drinks and asked if we were ready to order, thankfully he just let me choose, which was perfect. Expertly, I reeled off our order and he seemed content with my choices. So, we got back to talking about him. He barely asked me anything – except to find out the name of the most famous person I'd ever met. I knew it wasn't really a question for me to answer – he just wanted me to ask him the same thing. So I did, and he proceeded to tell me that he'd dined with the Beckhams and Jamie Oliver, and that David Beckham was really a lovely, genuine guy.

He then said, 'Tell me about you.' I hate it when people say that – it's such a cop-out when they should be the one asking the questions, generally showing an interest. 'What do you want to know?' I asked. 'Whatever you want to tell me,' he said – another cop-out. He wasn't really interested in me he just thought he ought to ask. I tried to sound enthusiastic, telling him about my family and background, but he didn't ask one question so it soon fizzled out and we got back to talking about him. I really wasn't surprised that he was single! 'I've also met Princess Diana' blah, blah… Eager to get the conversation away from him, I jumped at the opportunity to ask if he believed in any of the Diana conspiracy theories. That's the kind of conversation I find interesting. If someone is 'me, me, me', it's just boring.

We had a leisurely dinner and after I'd polished off my food and had a mint tea, he asked if I wanted anything else and what time we had left. It was now gone 11.30p.m., so I said we had about an hour. He asked if I minded going to the room, which I thought was very polite of him. 'Of course not,' I said, with a smile and a twinkle in my eye, and we both stood up to go. When we reached the room, he confided in me that he'd forgotten to bring protection and apologised for embarrassing me. I told him I'd come prepared and had my box of tricks.

In the bathroom, I took my tights off while he lit the candles. When I came out, he said he'd lit them but they'd all blown out with the air con. The lights in the room were so bright, like big spotlights right over the pillows, which didn't make for a very romantic, sexy ambience. In my heels I was taller than him, so I bent down to kiss him and he pressed his erection against me. I reached down and rubbed it through his trousers as it pushed, wanting to be released.

Within a couple of minutes, we were naked and on the bed, the big spotlights shining in our eyes. He clasped his mouth around one of my breasts and then sucked them both in turn before moving between my legs for a few minutes; he then came back up and lay on his back for me to pleasure him. I licked up his shaft and took the head in my mouth; I could tell it wouldn't be long before he came. After a few seconds, he muttered that he was going to come – just as I was reaching up to kiss him, to hopefully prolong his erection.

It was too late, and as I lay on top kissing him, his member squashed between my breasts, I could feel him pumping out his come. I didn't move, and we lay and chatted for about 30 minutes, stuck together with me yawning as my beauty sleep beckoned. I stayed 15 minutes longer, before saying my thanks and goodbyes. He seemed happy and implied that he wanted to meet again. He was going to settle down to some work and I was off home to the land of nod after a relaxing bath.

CHAPTER 21:

Escort Etiquette

So, what do I expect from a date? Well, here's my general guide to escort etiquette.

Do:
- Treat the lady as a lady, not a sex object.
- Treat the lady with respect. It's not your right to see her it is her choice to see you.
- Offer her a drink when she arrives.
- Pay the lady without prompting, within ten minutes of her arrival.
- Consider her comfort above your own. It's an escort's job to make their date feel comfortable, and the more comfortable she is, the more comfortable she will make you.
- Let the lady set the pace. An experienced, good escort will move the meeting on at her pace, taking into consideration guy's needs and personalities.
- Be patient when waiting for a response. So many guys don't remember to leave their full name and phone number, but

they also forget we can sometimes be away for a few days. It's fine to follow up calls and emails, as long as you don't get obsessive.

- Read all the information you can about the escort. We are all very different and work very differently, so no experience will ever be the same. Some ladies sell sex and some sell companionship. It's imperative to do your homework first, so read all the reviews available as this will give you an idea what to expect. A good escort site will be informative and tell you about an escort's personality.
- Discuss any expectations or specific requirements regarding the date in advance, to prevent disappointment. For example, if a guy specifically wants to have multiple sex sessions on an overnight date, he needs to check that the escort will be OK with this. I'm a one-session-a-night girl: for me it's quality, not quantity.
- Make sure you are freshly showered and shaved, and smelling fresh.

Don't:
- Try to French kiss or grope an escort on arrival – it's considered extremely rude. You're unlikely to get the best out of her if you put her back up from the start. If a lady does this to you (it does happen), and you're uncomfortable, say you'd like to get to know her first.
- Ask personal questions or want to know about the guys she sees. Personally, I find it extremely patronising when people assume I meet idiots. It's insulting for them to think I would put up with being treated badly.
- Ask questions that are already answered on the lady's website. I get asked 'How much is it?' by people who claim to have read my site.
- Book a lady purely based on her looks. To save disappointment and wasting time and money, it's worth taking the time to find out if she can offer you the experience

you're after. The more explicit the site is, the more you can assume the meeting is about the sex. If there's little reference to sex and no explicit photos, don't assume you can request or expect a PSE.

- Repeatedly call, but never leave a message. It's a sign of an obsessive nature and I know I avoid people who always call without leaving a message. If it's not convenient, your call won't be answered, no matter how many times you try. We all have personal lives and it's not always convenient to answer a phone call. I always think email is a good first step, as long as you're booking a week or so in advance. Don't rely on emails, though, because they can go missing, so if you don't get a reply, it's worth following it up with a voicemail. I like to hear someone's voice before I decide whether to speak to them, so I often let my phone go to answer machine.

- Approach an escort if you see her out and about, regardless of whether you have seen her before. If you've met her before, it's OK to catch her eye and see how she responds. If she wants to, and is able to talk, then she will. She may appear to be on her own, but she could be waiting for friends or family, or have a boyfriend, husband or child nearby. Think if you are married how you'd feel being approached by an escort if you were maybe waiting for your wife outside a shop.

- Ask for discounts. It's extremely rude! You won't get the best out of an escort if you try to haggle. Guys need to find an escort within their budget. Never contact one that isn't, and then try to haggle.

- Be selfish and assume you can book a lady all night and not take her out of the room or feed her. I'd be off like a shot, so I do always check that we're going out before arranging overnight dates. I also expect to be fed in the morning before I leave, especially if I have a long journey home. Some guys assume their escort won't want breakfast just because they don't. Again, the more thoughtful a guy is, the more he will get out of a date.

- Book an escort if you think there's a chance you may have to cancel. Sometimes guys book multiple escorts in case unreliable ones cancel on them. We don't take kindly to being messed around. In my opinion, anyone decent should compensate the lady for the inconvenience if they have to cancel. Girls do let guys down too, and that's why guys should read the reviews and research properly before making a choice.

- Expect to become 'friends' once you've met a lady. I'm not escorting to make friends, so being contacted by guys looking for friends, with or without arranging a paid date, is not acceptable. Most escorts have busy lives and we simply don't have the time to maintain friendships with everyone we see.

- Call during unsociable hours. I don't return any calls left during unsociable hours; it tells me a lot about someone's personality. I prefer weekday calls from 9–5, but everyone is different. It's worth looking on the escort's website and seeing whether she mentions a good time to call. If she doesn't, I'd say that between 9a.m. and 10p.m. is acceptable. Also, I wouldn't call on a Sunday or public holiday unless you want to meet that day.

- Try to stay longer than the hours you've paid for, unless the escort initiates it. Some guys try and take the piss by tilting the alarm clock so the time isn't visible, hoping we'll get lost in the moment.

Diary: September 2008

As I plucked the chocolate body sauce pen from the hanger in Ann Summers, a devilish smile played on my lips. I imagined how I was going to treat Tom for his birthday, drawing 'Happy birthday Tom' across my body for him to lick off. I'd also said I'd give him a £300 discount as a birthday gift.

My mind whirred as I thought about what else I would need for his birthday surprise. I scanned the rows of lingerie and my eyes settled on a short, sheer lace skirt and panties combo. It was crotchless, not that that would be much use as Tom never touches me down below, but I liked the skirt. Next to it was a rail of hold-up black stockings with small red bows, and I grabbed a pair.

I imagined the completed outfit, with my Agent Provocateur nipple tassels (a present from my gay friends), the birthday message on my body, the skirt and panties with stockings, and some killer platform heels. I thought I might also get him a little birthday cake with a candle. My friend Keith rang while I was shopping and I told him about my little plan. 'You didn't do that for my birthday!' he said. 'Well, you didn't pay me £500!' I replied, teasing him.

My date with Tom was last night. For a change I'd booked us into an Indian restaurant and we made our way there shortly after I arrived. He'd watched the footie and his team had lost, so he needed a bit of cheering up. We ate and chatted for the next three hours, before retiring to the room. It was freezing! I needed to warm the place up before I contemplated getting naked, so we put the heater on. Tom always brings an extra heater and a T-shirt for me to wear, as he likes me leaving my smell on his shirt. Unfortunately, his heater wouldn't work. He fiddled with it, with me moaning how cold it was. I used the hair dryer to try and warm myself up. Eventually, we worked out that it would be warmer to keep the hotel's heater off, as it was blowing cold air instead of warm.

I banished him to the bathroom as I set about the task of writing with the chocolate body paint. It looked like a child's writing, and I was making a right mess and getting it everywhere. As I bent down to put on my platform heels, I smudged the writing. Oooops! I was about to add the nipple tassels to complete the outfit, when I realised the 'h' and the 'y' were both around my nipples, so there was lots of chocolate on my boobs and the tassels didn't stick very well.

'Can I have a wank while I wait?' asked Tom, shouting through to me. 'No, you can't!' I exclaimed, 'I'm almost ready!' I got the little cake, lit the candle and then called him out. Cake in hand and covered in chocolate body sauce, I stood sexily, grinning away, and then launched into 'Happy birthday' in my best Marilyn Monroe. He laughed delightedly, 'Ooo, Rach, you tease, you tease!' Then he stood back and admired my artwork. I explained it was edible chocolate, but after four courses at the Indian, I don't think he was quite hungry enough to lick it all off. 'Your tits look great, Rach!' he observed. 'I think they're bigger than last time.' I always fuel his fantasy by telling him that they feel bigger, so I agreed with him.

He licked the bits off my boobs, and ended up with chocolate all over his face and mouth, like a naughty little boy. Then, as I got the feeling he didn't want any more chocolate, I told him it was OK if he wanted to wipe the rest off, so that's what he did. 'Oooh! I think Percy likes it,' he said of his penis, as he admired the lingerie I had bought. Black is his favourite colour, so I usually wear black lingerie and sometimes black clothes, too. I lay on top of him, squishing my breasts into him. 'Oooh! That feels so nice, Rach,' he moaned. Our short session ended with Tom relieving himself between my breasts – he normally does this when we're together. It turns me on, so I quite enjoy our little sessions. It wasn't long before little Percy could bear it no longer and he shot his load. Off he went to the bathroom to get a wet flannel to clean me up.

He then pulled out the sofa bed, I slapped a snore strip on him and we both settled to sleep. I'd met him at 7.30 and it was now midnight. I was the first to stir at 8am, and I listened to him snoring loudly for the next 30 minutes before popping my head up as he opened his eyes. 'Where be my Tom to?' I joked. 'I be here,' he replied.

He got up, put the bed away and jumped in with me. Percy wasn't playing this morning, so I gave up on it and put the kettle on instead. We sat and had tea before I left him to it. I think he appreciated his little birthday treat!

CHAPTER 22:

The Kinky Jobs

I've had some odd requests in my time. Once, I was asked if I was ready for a new type of sexual experience, money no object. Even though I knew it was going to be something dodgy, curiosity got the better of me. I asked the guy in question exactly what it would involve, and was informed that I would stay with him on his boat in the Caribbean, which he shared with his 'darlings' – five Bonobo chimpanzees – and a doctor. He didn't actually ask me to have sex with them, but he insisted they were very well looked after and everything was very safe, so it was obvious what he was implying. Needless to say, I didn't go!

Another strange request came when I had just started escorting and wasn't an expert in dealing with calls, especially unusual ones. I had a call from a mother, who said she wanted me to have sex with her 15-year-old daughter while she watched. She even put her 'daughter' on the phone, and it did sound like a young girl. I was totally freaked out and didn't know what to say – if I'd had any suspicion this was a serious request, I would have called the police, but it was obviously a wind-up, so I just put the phone down.

Most men like some form of anal play, with fingers and vibrators, and I guess that's considered kinky by some. I've experimented with it with boyfriends. They've all professed to hate the idea (some men have the misguided view that getting pleasure from anal might mean they're gay), but eventually, with a little gentle persuasion, they've all loved it! With work it's not something I do as a rule, but very occasionally, if I'm in the mood and they're ultra-clean, I will do rimming and have a probe with my fingers. One guy mentioned this 'thing' that some girls had done that he really liked, but said other girls had tried it and it wasn't very good as their technique was all wrong. He said it was something one of his favourite escorts had introduced him to. I guessed that it was the finger in the ass, but he wouldn't say exactly what he was talking about, so I decided to tease it out of him.

After about five minutes, we both stripped down to our underwear and I straddled him. He removed my bra and seemed pleased with what was underneath. We then moved side by side, and he asked what I thought the girls he'd seen had said the best part of his body was. Straightaway, I said his bum. I think he was surprised that I got it right! I said, 'Come on then, let's take a look,' prompting him to turn onto his front. I admired and squeezed his ass, and agreed it was very nice. Then I removed his underpants and gently parted his legs. I licked and kissed between his thighs and ran my finger between his bum cheeks, before sliding my boobs over his bum, up his back and then back down again.

Feeling particularly naughty, I reached for my lube and squeezed the tube above the crack of his bum, where it dripped between his cheeks. I then used my fingers to smooth it over his bum-hole and over his balls, and reached between his legs to smooth it over his penis. He was groaning and I could tell he really wanted me to insert my finger into his hole. His bum was getting more raised as he pushed it towards me, urging me on, and also giving me space to play with his penis at the same time. I licked his bum and teased my fingers around it, all the time alternating between his bum, balls and penis, now sticky and wet with lubrication. This allowed me to keep the movements fluid and my hands and fingers slid easily between them.

I then started probing his hole with my finger, while masturbating him with my other hand. I could tell he was close to coming. I hadn't even given him oral sex and I still had my pants on. One finger was inserted into him, the other masturbating him. I could tell he was about to come as his groans got louder and eventually he turned on to his back and came all over my body. I know he was blown away by the experience because he said how amazing it was, so I'm confident I will be seeing him again.

The fun jobs are the two-girl ones. I realised when I was in primary school that I was bisexual, when I tempted a girl into my bed. We were about eight years old, and I knew it was naughty, but it excited me. I'd tell her that she could touch me if I could touch her. Since then, I'd had various experiences with other girls but didn't have sex with another woman until a couple of years before I started escorting. I met her through my boyfriend at the time and he knew her boyfriend because they were both paratroopers.

We got drunk one night at a party and she and I ended up in the shower together, then all four of us went to bed. The lads watched us girls play with each other and then we had sex with our respective partners. It was a new experience for me and it was great fun.

Generally speaking, I save fantasy and role play for boyfriends, but I've done a couple of role plays for work. One guy wanted me to pretend that he was a teacher. This was a two-girl job, with my young 18-year-old friend, and we both had to dress up in school uniform. When I wear a school uniform I feel naughty and something comes over me (no, not like that!) – I just switch into the role very easily. At college, I would get told off for running around the corridors whenever I had my school uniform on! The guy we met was in his fifties and looked very much like a teacher. We giggled like schoolgirls and I was trying to blame my friend, so she'd get into trouble. He accused us of smoking and said he'd tell our parents unless we performed certain sexual acts on him. I loved it – it was fun and exciting, especially with my friend being there too.

The best schoolgirl fantasy I had was meeting a client of mine, Robert, who is also a close friend. He looks very much like a teacher. He's in his fifties and is attractive, with silver hair. We met at the Baglioni for an overnight date, and the role play started at dinner. In the restaurant, the tables were literally inches away from each other. He started saying, 'Well, I need to speak to you about some inappropriate behaviour...' I giggled nervously, but felt excited at the same time. There was a couple sitting just a few inches away from us and I saw their ears prick up. Robert looked very stern, and I found it very sexy. He proceeded to pull out some photographs of me that he had taken from my website. I hadn't expected him to go to so much trouble! He handed them to me, one by one, asking, 'And what's the meaning of this?' There I was, sitting on the floor in white panties and pink pigtails, with my knees together, but legs apart so my slit was visible through my panties. He'd superimposed a photo of some teenagers in school uniform into the background, which he'd found on a website that offered free images. It looked really funny. 'Oh, I... er...' I didn't know what to say. I just giggled nervously and said, 'Oh, it's nothing.' 'And what about this?' he asked, while pulling another photo of me out of his jacket pocket. I came up with pathetic excuses and he chastised me for my 'inappropriate behaviour'.

The quiet couple beside us didn't know what to make of the

situation. Robert was so good at the role play – he appeared to be deadly serious. We kept it up for the whole meal before he said that he wanted to have words with me in private, upstairs in the room, and that I was in very big trouble. The couple's faces next to us were hilarious. They barely spoke to each other during their meal and I'm sure they were listening to every word! Both glanced over as he pulled out the photos! I could tell the guy was probably very envious of this saucy couple next to him. Back in the room I put on my uniform and my punishment was to perform various acts on him.

On another date Robert took me to Spearmint Rhino. The dancers make a bee-line for ladies who are part of a couple. I find it extremely erotic to watch women pole dance and to receive a lap dance. When I've been with boyfriends or other men, I tend to find that they get off on watching your facial expressions during the dance as much as looking at the dancer themselves. He really treated me that night – I was allowed to pick a girl for a dance. We got approached by many girls but they weren't trying to make any effort at conversation – it was just a bored-sounding, 'Do you want a dance?' Each time we declined, until two dancers came and sat with us, and actually made an effort. We then both enjoyed a lap dance at the same time, glancing and smiling at each other.

After the ladies left, another girl approached and showed interest in me; she asked if I'd like a private dance and he said if I'd like one, he'd pay. So, he gave her the money and she took me by the hand into a private booth. She looked me in the eye and started stripping off, her eyes constantly staying on mine, teasing me. She stood up and purposely brushed her nipple across my mouth and the smooth skin of her breast across my cheek, all the time writhing away to the music. Then she bent over in front of me so that her crotch was inches from my face. This was my foreplay! Robert had already said that when we got back to the hotel, I could book a lady of my choice for an hour. By the time the dance was over, I was ready for some fun.

We left, and back in the room we got out his laptop and started browsing the Internet for bisexual escorts. I suppose it's bizarre that you can buy people for a certain amount of time. It was surreal, and I'd never really thought about it before – I'd never looked at escort sites with the view to booking anyone. It was just like ordering a takeaway, only way more satisfying! I think one way to tell if a lady is truly bi is if she's willing to give oral sex to women. I've been with girls before who just use toys, or expect you to do everything to them; they're the ones I don't think are bi. So we called an agency and asked who was genuinely bisexual; an Eastern European lady was recommended. She was tall, dark and had a lovely body. We booked her for an hour, and didn't mention that I was an escort.

We had around an hour to wait before her arrival, so we ordered a bottle of champagne. I'd been on jobs with other girls before, but nobody had actually let me book a lady, so I was really excited. This was different as it wouldn't feel like 'work' to me; I knew she'd be the one doing her 'job', and although I was booked for the evening, it would be different as it felt like Robert and I were a real couple, booking an escort. Eventually the agency called to say she was downstairs, so I made my way down to collect her. I felt nervous; it was a strange, unfamiliar feeling for me.

As I stepped out, she was waiting by the lift. She was so tall and beautiful, with pale skin and dark wavy hair, just like her photos. I kissed her hello and guided her back up in the lift. She stood grinning at me in a naughty way as the lift went up, as if to say, 'I'm going to ravish you once we get in that room!' Her sexuality radiated off her and I found my heart was hammering in my chest.

We got to the room and I let her in. Robert introduced himself – this was all so normal to him, but so different for me. From the start it was clear she was a pro. Her English wasn't good, which made for minimal conversation as she perched on the end of our huge bed. She had a small glass of champagne, which she finished quickly, and declined a top-up – she was obviously keen to get things going. I'd imagined that we'd all be together as a cosy threesome, but she saw me and Robert as two individuals wanting to be serviced individually, which was fine by me! Threesomes are fun, but I never orgasm as there's so much going on – trying to look after two people means I can't relax enough to orgasm unless I use my toy.

It seems she was a traditionalist like me, as it was 'ladies first'. She'd slipped off her tight jeans, boots and sexy blouse, leaving her with gorgeous black lace lingerie on a toned body. She didn't even look at Robert as she crawled up to me, kissing me softly and undressing me, until I was left exposed and naked. Robert watched us curiously, undressing, but all the time watching her, leaving just his boxer shorts on. He settled back and lay down. Her attention was on me; this was my time, his turn would come. She gently stroked and kissed my body like she had all the time in the world. I was so horny, especially after my private dance. The thing I love about women is their soft, gentle and sensuous touch. Men can be too cumbersome with their eagerness and their big, rough, excitable hands.

After only a few minutes she was licking me down below, ever so softly, but consistently. It usually takes me a long time to come – if I even come at all – but this woman knew what she was doing. Robert watched, intrigued and excited, waiting his turn. I closed my eyes and allowed myself to fully relax and savour the moment. She made me orgasm and it was the quickest I think I've ever come. I was totally blown away by the experience, panting for air with a contented smile on my face.

Straightaway, she turned her attention to Robert, as I lay immobile, flushed and glowing, grinning like a Cheshire cat. Robert doesn't like condoms and usually I struggle to make him come, so even though we have sex, we finish up with oral.

I can feel him start to lose his erection as soon as the condom's on. She, however, gave him oral sex for a short while, whacked a condom on in about a second and was immediately grinding back and forth on top. I was trying to watch and learn as she rode him to a climax in less than five minutes. How the hell did she do that? What a pro! I remember thinking that I could sure use some tips from her. She left after 40 minutes, even though we had paid for an hour, but we were both satisfied and went to sleep with smiles on our faces.

Assignments with other girls are usually fun especially when it's someone you know and can have a laugh with. I once met Lisa (a friend I know through work) with one of her regulars for his birthday treat. The plan was to have dinner and then go clubbing because Jim loves to dance. Lisa was arriving in Manchester first, and then I was to join them later. Lisa isn't bi as she doesn't give ladies oral sex, but we do have fun when we work together. I remember being in the shower, doing my normal pre-work routine of shower, shave and nails, when suddenly I remembered Lisa would be there and that we were going clubbing, which made me smile to myself. It would just be like a night out, especially as Lisa and I get on so well and have such a laugh together. It just meant there was sure to be sex at the end of the night – she wanted to treat her date to some birthday fun!

On my journey, Lisa and I were texting each other. She'd forgotten to bring tampons, but I had already left so I couldn't get any. I had a couple with me – it was the time of the month for both of us! What a coincidence. Oh well, thank God for natural sponges! This is one of our tricks of the trade. You put a bit inside you, just before you have sex, and you can't feel it, and neither can the guy, but it does the job of a tampon very well. It can be fiddly to get out, but it's worth it.

A taxi dropped me off by this huge apartment complex. Lisa came to find me, and we bumped into each other by the lifts. Giggling, we got the lift together. When Lisa got to the room we were still giggling as she rapped on the door. 'Room service!' she hollered, and 'Jim Bobitty Bob,' which is her nickname for him. I was laughing my head off, and after about five minutes, when we realised there was no answer, I looked at the room numbers and realised we were on the wrong floor! Mortified, we both started cracking up again and I knew the night would be fun. When we got to the right floor, I hid and Lisa walked in with my case. Then Jim came out onto the landing, and was genuinely shocked to see me – he didn't know what to expect for his birthday treat. He cracked open the pink champagne I had brought with me and we toasted his birthday in style!

We ate at an Italian restaurant before heading straight for the club. After a couple of vodkas I wanted to have a snog with Lisa, so I loomed in for a kiss. Jim joined in too, and we all sat in a three-way snog for ages, while I was reaching under Lisa's dress and playing with her panties. Soon we were all up dancing, Jim sandwiched between us. He looked like the cat that got the cream, which I suppose he was!

We could see younger, fitter men glancing over and wondering how the hell he'd managed to pull us both. I remember that when I was younger and didn't know about escorts, I used to be just as confused, but since I've become one I can look at men and women together and am able to spot them. Even in lifts, when a lady walks in on her own, I can usually tell if she's an escort. Maybe it's the air of confidence, together with the smart clothes, immaculate make-up and nails, plus expensive bag and the fact that they're in the lift on their own that makes me assume they're off to see a client. Escorts stride into hotels confidently, and try to discreetly suss out where the lifts are. Sometimes I will be on the phone to my client as I enter a hotel and he will actually talk me through the layout and point me in the right direction. Being on the phone is a good distraction, anyway – hotel staff don't tend to pay much attention to people on mobile phones.

Anyway, back to my saucy night out... All these men were just gawping at us, and Lisa and I were pawing all over Jim, leaning over him for a snog with each other. Then I pressed myself up behind Lisa so she was sandwiched in, and we were all grinding away and groping each other. I have to admit that Lisa and I do make a good couple, because we are so different. We're both about the same height, but she has dark hair and dark skin. Her waist is tiny, but she has large boobs and a peachy bum, which gives her the perfect hourglass figure, while I am blonde and fair-skinned, with smaller boobs, but I'm in proportion.

After a good few hours we all linked arms and left the club. We made our way back to our apartment block and tumbled straight into the bedroom. Lisa and I went to the bathroom and showered, while giggling about putting sponges in. She used a 'Rammer' sponge, so I was laughing at the name (it's a brand of man-made sponges that are soft when wet, but hard when dry), because she couldn't get it in. So I sat on the loo and she put one leg up on the side and I just rammed it in. I'm surprised Jim stayed awake – we must have been giggling in the shower for about 20 minutes!

Eventually we came out and we started playing. Jim was extremely excited as he'd been waiting for this moment all night! All his clothes were quickly ripped off and we got straight down to business, tongues and dangly bits everywhere. Jim went down on Lisa and I asked if I could have a go, so we took it in turns. He then put a condom on and pumped away at Lisa. He didn't come, and then he tried with me and still didn't manage it. In the end I suggested he finished himself off, and Lisa and I lay there, begging him to come on our naked bodies! This was all the prompting he needed to finish the job.

I've seen real couples before, but generally I don't enjoy it because often the lady is only doing it to please her man, and it's clear that she feels extremely uncomfortable. I always insist on speaking with her first to check she's OK with things, but still women will say they are, just to please their men.

I once went to meet a couple for a dinner date and when we moved to the bedroom, the guy was ordering his girlfriend to go down on me and she didn't want to. She was embarrassed and uncomfortable, and so was I. He rather selfishly didn't care and kept asking her, while I was asking him to stop pressurising her. It was awful! You have to have a very special relationship to be able to bring in a third party. Both people have to be extremely secure with themselves as individuals and as a couple.

I once met a wonderfully eccentric couple, Charles and Vivian, and had an amazing time with them. The lady called, which impressed me. She was very well-spoken and explained that she and her and her husband were in their fifties; she said she was attractive and did yoga, and then went on to say they had never done anything like this before, but they both wanted the experience. She wanted to have sex with another woman, and her husband wanted to watch that too, and she wanted to watch me with her husband. There were no restrictions on what I could and couldn't do. It was his birthday present – what a cool wife, eh?

It was arranged that they would travel up to Nottingham and we would all meet up for a dinner date. To make the right impression, I wanted to wear something classy and sophisticated. I chose my sheer La Perla lingerie and a simple black shift dress, which I jazzed up with some forties-style Fendi sandals and my dark red bag, which everyone assumes is expensive, but actually only cost £30! I finished off the look with my Tiffany chain necklace and some diamond earrings, both were presents from clients. It was a sexy outfit, but in an understated way.

I took a bottle of bubbly as a present for him, and some chocolates for her. I was very pleased when I saw her – the first thing I noticed was that she was a very stunning blonde. She had told me she was attractive, but I know sometimes people overrate themselves so it was a pleasant surprise! They both had a great sense of humour, and I loved their posh accents. It just made the whole thing seem naughtier! Charles was wearing a dark suit with a shirt and tie, while Vivian wore a black-and-white dress with a full skirt. We did all go together very well, clothes-wise, so I felt very comfortable and was pleased with my choice of dress. I was confident we would have a fun evening. Over dinner, Vivian started flirting with me and making suggestive comments to Charles about what we would get up to, much to the amusement of the waiting staff. I couldn't even concentrate on the delicious food – it was clear they had other things on their mind.

Back in the room, Vivian took the initiative and was eager to get things going. She and I undressed each other and kissed. She kept looking at her husband over my shoulder and saying, 'Do you like that, Charles? Do you like seeing me with Bea? Does it turn you on? It's turning me on.' Of course, he loved it! And her talk was exciting him more, as he was watching with keen interest and a solid erection. Then we both moved to the bed and took it in turns to kiss him, and then each other, while undressing him.

Vivian asked Charles if he'd like to watch her give me oral sex, which of course he did, so I lay down and she proceeded to lick me and probe my pussy. Then he watched as I returned the favour. I pulled out my vibrator and started using it on Vivian, first on the outside and then inside her as she groaned loudly and begged me to carry on. He was blown away by the whole experience. It was then his turn and Vivian and I both took turns to lick his cock, sometimes at the same time while holding his gaze. She then inquired very matter-of-factly if Charles would like to fuck me, which I thought very generous of her. I got a condom and sat on top of him. She sat next to me as I rode him, licking my nipples and urging me on. Then we swapped over, and she removed the condom and sat on top of him grinding away. I caressed and played with her boobs until he reached a loud, satisfying orgasm.

They were an amazing couple, and I'm disappointed that I only saw them the once. A few months later, they wanted me to visit them at their home, but it was clear they didn't want to pay the rate for an extended date, so I didn't go. I imagine they maybe moved onto swinging, which would be more appropriate if they didn't have the money to spend on escorts.

Diary: December 2007

'I've seen you out and about,' said my date. 'In fact, I saw you last week – you were driving a yellow car.' 'Oh,' I offered meekly, feeling extremely uncomfortable with being spotted in my day-to-day life. 'I also saw you in the San Carlos restaurant when I was out with friends – you were with an old man.' (That would have been John, my regular.) He then proceeded to tell me he'd seen me shopping and in various other places. OK, he was starting to freak me out now.

This is one of the drawbacks of having my face on the Internet. I'm bound to be recognised on occasion. Sometimes I see people staring at me and my first thought is always that they must recognise me from the Internet. There are other possibilities, of course – they may be staring at my beauty, or alternatively, as I'm not a stereotypically beautiful lady, maybe they're looking out of morbid curiosity. A small child once told me that I had a 'funny face', and by 'funny', it was clear she meant odd. You can trust innocent, honest children to say what they see! Then there's always the thought that I might have food on my face or a big spot.

My date was a good looking guy, which was rare. I'd thought initially that he was younger than me, but when he proceeded to talk about his company and his £800,000 tax bill for the year, I realised he was extremely successful and assumed he must be older. I had only been booked for two hours, but he was very relaxed and we sat drinking and chatting for over an hour. We spoke about the world today, the prison system, books, and he seemed in no rush to jump onto the bed. This is my ideal client: chilled. In fact, we talked so much that it was me who thought I ought to get things moving to a more intimate level.

I took the candles out of my bag of tricks, lit them and placed them around the room, while he went to the bathroom. Then, when I came out of the bathroom in my Aubade sheer nude and black lingerie set, he was lying on the four-poster. I smiled at him seductively and joined him; we lay kissing and caressing. His featherlike touch was highly erotic, and I could feel myself getting aroused. He moved between my legs and licked gently around my clitoris, while holding my arms to the side. Moments like that make me really love my job!

Eventually he lay back and I went to return the favour, licking between his legs and his balls. His appreciative groaning confirmed he was enjoying what I was doing. He spread his legs, opening himself up to me and encouraging me to lick further down towards his anus. I licked and teased, alternating between this and sucking his penis; first, at the top and swirling my tongue around, then taking it all in my mouth and combining this with fluid hand movements. He was watching me, getting turned on by me satisfying him in the candlelight.

I moved back up to kiss him while reaching for my bag to get a condom. 'Ouch!' he said, as I was putting it on. Geez, you'd think I'd be an expert at it by now! I cringed and apologised, then I sat on top of him, gently easing myself down on him. Both of us moved: him pushing up, me pushing down. I lay back and arched my back as he pushed upwards; it felt amazing. I leaned forward and he placed his hands on my collarbone to keep me upright so I could lean forward, while moving up and down.

We moved ourselves into the missionary position (which I think is so under-rated), and he pumped away until he came and collapsed on top of me. I wrapped my legs around him and held him tightly there for a few minutes before he went to dispose of the condom. It transpired that he was 28, single and had met a few bunny boilers in his time. One of them he had dated on three occasions. He'd left her in his house once with a spare key so that she could lock up. Then one day he came home from work to find her sitting in his lounge! She'd had a key cut from his spare, let herself in and waited for him, and then asked why he hadn't called her.

Seeing escorts, for him, was an easy way to avoid these complications. I would hardly be ringing him in a couple of weeks, asking why I hadn't heard from him! We got dressed and he headed out to meet his friends in a bar, while I went home for my beauty sleep.

CHAPTER 23:

Sex With an Ex

O ver the years, I've had some great jobs and sometimes I get a thrill from my work dates, but for me I only get real satisfaction when there's closeness in a genuine relationship. Its great fun and I love getting paid to go on dates, but if I'm single for a while, then I really start to miss that special connection.

I do crave that sort of connection, as most of my friends have a man or at least some sort of sexual excitement in their lives. For me, work doesn't count – I miss the closeness of being with someone I'm physically attracted to, and who I have an emotional relationship with. I don't want a one-night stand, because I find they're always a disappointment, and too much like work. Once I'd decided I wanted something to happen, it had to be with someone I already knew, because I was feeling very impatient. It'd been too long.

I started making a mental list of my male friends and exes, reminiscing about past times that had been good. It seemed that my only safe option was my first love, James. A great candidate!

I'd met up with him for drinks in London a couple of months before, and he was flirting with me. He would be a safe bet because there'd be no chance of me falling for him again, and I felt that I would still be comfortable with him because we were together so long. He's now 28, and I'm still physically attracted to him. So, one day, when I was in an impulsive mood, I sent him a text saying, 'When are you coming to Nottingham? Because I need some lovin'...' I got a text back: 'Are you serious? Would you like to see Doctor Love?' That's a role-play we used to enjoy when we were together; we'd take it in turns to play 'doctor'. It used to turn me on so much.

When he was pretending to be a doctor he would leave me lying on the bed at his house while his parents were out. About ten minutes later, he would knock on the door – by this time I was so excited and turned on by the thought of what was going to happen. When he entered the room, he'd have improvised and dressed up. He'd look all serious, carrying a clipboard and pen, and he'd be wearing glasses. He looked such a geek but it turned me on because I knew he was underneath. He was hot! He'd ask if I was 'Miss X'. Grinning, I'd confirm that I was. Then we proceeded to role play, with him inspecting me and having to do things to me to make me better. He changed his voice and really got into his role, and by the time we had sex, I was so turned on!

Anyway, so we went back and forth with text banter and I lost track of the time, caught up in my memories. On the way to the supermarket, I decided to ring him when I was in the car. I told him I really wanted him to do me this favour and fuck my brains out. He was taken aback and I knew he was wondering if I was joking. I told him I hadn't had sex for ages, and that work didn't count, and that I didn't want a one-night stand with a stranger; I wanted to be with someone I was comfortable with. I asked him when he could fit me in for an appointment, and he said he had a hard-on, thinking about it, and that he would come up as soon as he could. I ended up going to the supermarket with a big grin on my face and couldn't remember when I'd been that excited about anything! I felt liberated, it was very odd.

The next morning I get a text message from James: 'I am looking at your pictures on your website and wanking over you. You look so sexy!' A big smile creeps across my face and I very quickly type back, 'send me a piccie, you dirty boy!' Within seconds, a naked photo comes through... a little bit too quickly, I think, for it to have just been taken! I'm thinking it was saved in his phone and he sends it out to girls he's messing around with. He says there's only one, but James always has been a compulsive liar! The text reads: 'I am gonna fuck you good baby.'

I get a warm tingly feeling down below; I feel so horny. I can't believe how exciting all this is! I spend ages trying to take a nice picture of myself. I decide to stand on my tiptoes, naked, and take one in the mirror. I'm very pleased with the result – you can't really see my face because it's quite dark, but I look tall and slim because I'm on my tiptoes, and it's a good body shot, without being explicit. So, I send it through as a text with, '.... Waiting for you XXX.'

He eventually texted back to say that he didn't think it was a good idea as we had only just got back to being friends. I was totally gutted after all that build-up and excitement! It was so typical of him, after he had teased me into sending him that photo. I don't expect to hear from him for a while. It can be great texting someone you really like, because you can be whoever you want to be in that moment. We had our bit of excitement, but needless to say, James didn't come to see me and I was disappointed.

I did recently go out on a non-work date, though, and it came about after a night out with my friend Katie G. One evening, we ended up at an extremely dodgy bar. As soon as I walked in, one guy's eyes almost popped out of his head. I didn't fancy him, but it was really quite flattering, though I felt a bit awkward because he wouldn't stop staring at me. I went to the bar to get our drinks and the guy staring at me was standing at the bar, so I just said 'Hi' to him. We started talking and he turned out to be really interesting. He was slightly taller than me and dressed very casually. It turned out that he was a quarter Chinese, a quarter Spanish and half-Jamaican. He had a definite Spanish look, but with Afro-Caribbean features.

At first, he thought that one of the guys we'd come in with was my boyfriend! Then I got the annoying, 'So, why haven't you got a boyfriend?' line. I absolutely hate that! I gave my standard answer: 'Because I haven't found anyone I consider decent enough to be my boyfriend!'

He was my age, and had many interests, including chess, martial arts, painting and horse riding. I remember thinking he was a bit of a geek, but I was enjoying talking to him. His name was Kenneth, and he said he preferred to be called that, rather than Ken or Kenny... Yes, definitely, geek alert! He said he liked to try new things and I listened intently as he spoke about his painting and how he'd put some of his nudes in a gallery and received commissions from a nude he'd painted. He introduced me to his friends, and eventually they decided they wanted to move on to a club, so off we went! It was there that he said he'd like to take me on a date.

If I meet a guy I like, then I never tell him I'm an escort. Not to be sneaky, but because I don't want to be judged. I want them to get to know me for me, though I would never enter into a sexual relationship without telling the guy first what I did. Before now, when I've told guys what I do for a living, they've asked how much it is to talk to me. I know they're only joking, but I find it extremely annoying. It's as if they don't know how to act around me: they look at me as though I've just grown a second head, or I'm a newly discovered species. 'I've never met an escort before,' they usually say. I suppose it's a bit of an unusual job.

Guys also then assume I'm working; that I'm out looking for punters on a Saturday night while drinking with my friends! Once, when I was out with my friends, a guy that I was interested in found out from someone that I was an escort, and he turned around to me and said that he wasn't about to pay for sex! It was unbelievable. Another time, I was at a party and sharing a taxi with a couple I'd met that evening. When I suggested we went outside five minutes early so that someone else didn't steal our cab, the guy said, 'Why, do you want to try and tout for some business?' It's extremely frustrating the way some people act with me, and the things they say sometimes.

Anyhow, Kenneth called a couple of days later, and I was taken aback by how soft and ladylike his voice was. We were due to meet for a date in about a week's time, but in the meantime, my friend let me down at the last minute for a Dolly Parton concert in Manchester. So, I had a mad panic on, trying to find someone to go with. As it was a midweek concert, which involved having to leave at 3.30p.m. and maybe not getting back until about 1am, I couldn't find anyone who was free. I texted Kenneth and asked what time he finished work. When he texted back to say that he was off work, I decided I would give him a call and ask if he wanted to join me. He was very excited and said he'd love to go.

The day we were due to meet I got this text message through: 'Ure mission, if you accept! Meet with target at train station and infiltrate. Beware the man is well versed in all arts of charm, entertainment and seduction! X'. I cringed, thinking, 'Oh dear – what have I let myself in for?'

When I arrived at the station and got out of my taxi, I thought I caught a glimpse of him inside, but I felt a bit self-conscious so I walked in a different entrance and tried to call him. It was him: he waved and made his way over. On the train, we talked for the whole journey about his family and his musical background. He's in a pop band and a rock band.

Even though I had said it took a lot to impress me, I found myself constantly saying that I was impressed (that's if it was all true). I mean, with the bands, the martial arts, chess, horse riding, painting... and then I also found out that he enjoyed karaoke, scuba diving, quiz nights and Gospel church! Then he told me he was writing two books, one of which was a very complex thriller. I was unsure whether he was a genuine person, but only time would tell.

We talked briefly about past relationships, and he told me he was shocked when I had said I wasn't going to shag him. He hated the word 'shag', suggesting that there were so many other nicer ways to put it, and that 'shagging' was not something he did. He implied he liked to make love to women, and give them pleasure. It was almost like he was saying the things he thought women wanted to hear! I asked him who he thought he was – Mr Lover-Lover? I know he realised I was very cynical when it comes to men and their motives.

He was very much the gentleman and when I was cold, he put an arm around me – although maybe it was just an excuse to touch me. There I go, being cynical again! We got our tickets and made our way into the concert. He was very excitable. Afterwards, we didn't have to wait long for our taxi. I had already made it clear to the driver that there were two drops, one at my place and then one at his. When I got home, Kenneth sent me a text message to say he'd had a fun evening. I wondered what he would say when I broke it to him what I do for a living!

I think it's hard for men to understand how I can jump into bed with total strangers for work, but then not do so in my personal life. The thing is, work is work, but although I sometimes enjoy it, it doesn't engage my emotions or my mind. I want any sex and intimacy outside work to mean something, to be with someone special.

When Friday came, I texted Kenneth and said I hoped he wasn't expecting to get his leg over that evening. He replied

SEX WITH AN EX

that, however hard I might find it to believe, there were still some decent men around, if I wanted to hang about to find out. Still very wary, I was intrigued to get to know him. I pulled up in my taxi and my driver pointed at Kenneth and asked if he was my date. I said he was, and he asked if he was wearing a dicky bow. I couldn't stop giggling, because he was – he was pacing up and down outside one of the dodgiest pubs in Nottingham wearing a suit and a bow tie! I crossed the road to meet him and he looked really nervous. I couldn't stop grinning at him. He greeted me and pecked me on the cheek, before discreetly putting his arm around me. He said he'd been waiting there for half an hour and he was freezing!

He took me to a place I hadn't been before – Tonic. We went up to the restaurant, which looked really cool; I was sure the food was going to be good, too. There, we sat down on a sofa and a guy came over to take our drinks order. Kenneth whispered that there should be some champagne already on ice – apparently he'd asked them just to bring it over without him having to say anything and I could tell he was disappointed they hadn't. It was a very thoughtful touch and totally unexpected. Yes, I was definitely impressed. Over drinks, he confided that he used to be a stripper, but had then found God. What an earth would he think of my job then?

I found him very interesting to talk to, so I decided to drop the bomb and asked if he was open-minded. He said that he was, and asked me why; I asked him what he thought I did. It turned out that he and his friends had been coming up with all sorts of ideas, from prostitute to stripper. I told him I was an escort, and he didn't look surprised. He said that he'd thought it was strange when the indiscreet taxi driver coming back from Manchester had mentioned that he'd taken me down to London for a few hours! I asked him what he thought an escort did – there was no way I wanted to lie to him. He said he thought that an escort went out to functions. I agreed, but said there was more to it than that, and told him that although it wasn't the main focus of my job, there was usually sex involved.

I couldn't read what he was thinking. I asked him if he thought any less of me and he said he didn't, but I wasn't sure if he meant it. Then I asked him if he found it strange that I don't sleep around in my personal life, yet I jump into bed for my job. He said not, which made me think that he must be a fake. I mean, what normal person wouldn't find that difficult to understand? I would!

I decided he must be a player and that I was just another challenge to him. Also, I wasn't sure if he understood my sense of humour as I like to take the piss out of myself and others. I love a bit of banter. I was teasing him about gaining and losing points when it came to impressing me. I seriously doubted he was being himself – I felt like I was getting his standard routine. Then I teased him some more about having a book on the art of seduction – and he was so tetchy about it that I'm sure I was right. I found it quite sad.

He settled the bill and we went off to find a bar, where he decided to try and read my palm. I said I didn't believe in that sort of thing and told him it was really cheesy, but he could do it if he wanted, as long as he told me something he wouldn't have been able to know any other way. Realising that I wasn't going to be impressed he looked at my palm and said I had a good long lifeline, and that was as far as it went.

I subtracted a point for that, and he looked a bit put out, and said that he wasn't going to do it, if I was scoring him. It was just supposed to be a bit of fun. He said he'd written a song about me, and then he sang a bit adding my name in the lyrics. I'm sure he used the same song and changed the name of the girl! It was all getting a bit much and came across as sheer desperation. With the writing, the bands, the song, the chess, the art, the martial arts, the church, palm reading... he was trying too hard!

Then we went to a karaoke bar that I had never been in

before. It was a bit dingy and we were definitely overdressed. I started to feel quite tipsy and decided to make a quick exit before I embarrassed myself. We had just finished our drinks and I remember saying to Kenneth that I had to go, and within two minutes I was in a cab and off on my way home! I think I must have just pecked him on the cheek and dived into a cab, and afterwards I felt really bad because he'd put so much effort into the evening and I'd run off just like Cinderella.

But I soon discovered that people can go from hero to zero in less than a week. I had the most bizarre experience with him a few days later. I'd invited him round to watch a DVD and have a bite to eat; I decided I wouldn't put any make-up on, so that he could just see me as I was. After all, we were only watching a DVD! I was looking forward to a nice relaxed and chilled evening. The buzzer rang at 7p.m. on the dot, and I was horrified to see he was wearing a suit. I wondered if he had come straight from work, but I doubted it. Suddenly, I felt really self-conscious. There was me, in a hooded top, with jeans, slippers and no make-up, and there he was in a suit and tie, just to come round for a DVD. Immediately, I thought, idiot! The bow tie and suit was kind of cool on our night out, but this was ridiculous.

I let him in and at once apologised for my appearance. He said he'd been in the pub across the road because he'd arrived half an hour early (why?), and I took his jacket and hung it up. It was all very formal. He looked eager, almost wired. I'd seen that look before, the look of desperation that I sometimes see in my work, and it made me feel sick. He was almost standing on top of me and I was so shocked I didn't say anything, which is unusual for me.

I offered him a drink and he followed me to the kitchen, hovering in my personal space. I mentioned his suit, and he asked if I wanted him to take his tie off. I said yes, and he said that he didn't know how to. Pass me the sick bucket! He was standing ridiculously close me, blocking my exit, and asking me to take his tie off for him. Oh, please! I bustled past him, and said that he must know how to take his own tie off. He was still right on top of me, and I hated it. How could I have got him so wrong? He was cheesy beyond belief!

The eagerness in his eyes made me feel really uncomfortable, but then he said he felt nervous. I asked him why, but I could tell that it was because he obviously had other motives apart from just watching a film. I told him he looked like he was expecting something, and I said if he was waiting for me to strip his clothes off and take him to bed, he was sadly mistaken.

I know a lot of women say no and then give in, but I was straight with him and said that I just wanted to get to know him. By now, I could tell it was all an act – there were so many things about him that just didn't ring true. He was trying to be 'into' everything, and it was all so false

After we'd eaten, we went to watch the film. He sat right next to me, far too close; it made me feel really uncomfortable. Thankfully, after the film he said he had to go, because he was going to Turkey for a martial arts presentation. Whatever! He reckoned he wanted to retire in the next couple of years and that, aside from his job at the bank, he sold racehorses. Afterwards, I relayed the goings-on to a few friends, and the more I thought about it, the more I knew he was a bit weird. Thankfully, I never heard from him again.

While telling the story to my friend Keith, he just laughed and said that on a third date, he would definitely have thought he was 'in there', being asked round to my house. I just don't get it! I asked him whether he'd still think that if he'd been told nothing was going to happen, and he said that yes, he would probably still expect to end up having sex. Are men really that stupid?

CHAPTER 24:

Being Single Isn't So Bad After All! Sigh...

Recently I met up with James, my ex, in London when I was working for a few days. My job was for two nights, but the guy had business meetings all day, leaving me the time free, thankfully, to entertain myself. James was working in a bar and was free during the day. We met for a coffee, and then went to a restaurant, where he said he would treat me to lunch. I think that's the only time he's ever offered to take me out, even when we were dating!

We ordered, and while we waited for our food, he told me he was now single, and that he would like to sleep with me and that he still really fancied me. I'd kind of forgotten about having sex with him, but agreed to it in principle, at some point. He suggested we went back to his that day. Unbelievable! Absolutely not, I said. I was working, but I told him that in a few weeks we could properly arrange a night of passion. He told me he worried about me because of my job. It was lovely for him to be concerned, but I found it extremely patronising, considering I'm a very careful and sensible person, and he is not. I was due to meet him the other week and when I called, he said he'd woken up under someone's table after a drunken night and couldn't remember how he got there!

After a lovely meal, we got the bill and he suggested we pay half each. I smiled to myself – so much for my 'treat'! He was still making false promises. The idea of having sex with him was becoming less appealing. Because of how he was being, I didn't find him attractive at all – it just shows you how women generally need to be stimulated mentally before they can physically fancy someone.

We went to a bar for a few drinks. Knowing I would be drinking later, I stuck to soft drinks, but he kept trying to force me to have some alcohol. I stuck to my guns, however, and had cranberry juice. He then tried to be all 'couply' with me and put his arms around me; I really didn't feel comfortable. I got a call for work, and he asked me not to answer it. I didn't, but not because of him – I wanted to see if they left a message. He then tried to persuade me not to go back to my job, saying he would take the night off, if I did. Yeah right, I lose out on £1,000 and damage my reputation, and he loses out on £40 and keeps his job? Let me think about that one!

I couldn't bear to be with him any longer, so I said I had to go. He walked me back some of the way and left me at a shop that I wanted to browse in. We stood in the doorway and he went to kiss me goodbye. I pecked him, but he wanted a snog. There was no way I was going to do that in public, so I pecked him again and he went off in a sulk, saying that I wouldn't even give him a proper kiss. I remembered yet again what I'd had to put up with for all those years!

The most recent man that I slept with outside work was when I went to the Grand Prix in May last year. My friend and I met a bunch of guys in a bar in Monaco. They were all successful businessmen, aged between about 40 and 60 – the kind of guys I usually see for work. They were lovely guys and bought us

loads of drinks. By the end of the night we were quite tipsy and
they invited us to their boat, saying that we wouldn't get a taxi
home. My friend didn't want to go, but I managed to convince
her by organising for us to have a room to ourselves. The boat
had six bedrooms and was huge! In the morning, we both had
hangovers and stayed on the boat for breakfast. The guys then
suggested we stayed for the day while they were out at the
racing, so they went off, leaving us with passes to get back to
the port area.

We did a bit of shopping and then just sunbathed on the
deck. Eventually they came back on board and kindly asked us
to join them for dinner that evening. We'd bought a bottle of
champagne because we didn't want them to think we were
taking advantage, but when we presented it, one of the guys
said, 'I don't know why you bought this – we already have a
hundred bottles!'

Then one of them came up behind me, slipped his hands
around my waist and kissed me on the lips. I was taken aback
that he was so forward and instantly felt uncomfortable. Also,
I was racking my brains to work out whether I'd done
anything the night before to encourage that sort of intimacy.
I was tipsy, so I was struggling to remember, but then it came
back to me: he had tried to kiss me when we got back to the
boat, and I'd just gone with the flow and snogged him. For me,
that was quite full-on, not my usual behaviour outside of
work! Once you've crossed the barrier into the intimacy zone,
it's difficult to pull back and I silently cursed myself. He was
an extremely funny and charismatic guy, and if he hadn't
been such a fast mover, I know he would have definitely
grown on me.

I decided to switch into work mode, which was totally out
of character for me – I just accepted this was going to be the
deal, if we wanted to stay on the boat. It was very bizarre.
I knew I would end up sleeping with him and that it was my
choice, but I didn't really want it to happen – not because I

didn't like him, but because I didn't know him, so it felt like work.

That evening, my friend and I told the guys we were escorts. One guy's jaw just hit the floor! Apparently they'd had Brazilian hookers on the boat previously, and probably thought we didn't look like 'those' sort of girls, which of course we weren't (we weren't even looking for work!). We tried to explain how what we did was different since we both specialised in longer meetings and dates, and both offered the GFE.

I suppose, like most men, the guy I was with must have thought I was some kind of nymphomaniac because of my job. For the rest of the trip, I ended up sharing his room and I had sex with him, but it felt like it was expected of me. He expected me to perform for him to get his rocks off, yet I was getting nothing out of it at all.

Back in the UK, I met up with him a couple of times and explained how I thought we had rushed into things and it wasn't 'me' just to meet a guy and sleep with him. I told him the last guy I had slept with (because work doesn't count) was my ex, who I saw on and off for two years. It soon fizzled out anyway, though, because it turned out he was married and I have no interest in sleeping with a married guy unless I'm being paid.

Recently, I thought about seeing a male escort and trawled the Internet for a suitable candidate, but I couldn't quite find what I was looking for. Saying that, I also wasn't sure exactly what I wanted, but I came up with the following list:

- Reasonably good looking
- Nice, toned body, but not OTT body builder type
- Friendly face
- Someone with reviews would be nice, but there are no review sites for straight guys

- A guy who's 100% straight. I wouldn't want someone bi; it would need to be someone who loves ladies only.

In reality, while I find the whole idea intriguing, it's also bloody scary! My main fear is that they might fall short of my high expectations. The only promising candidate was Australian Ben – although he wasn't usually a type that I would go for in my personal life, he seemed to fit the bill. The only drawback was that he was listed on one of the sites as being bi. Most sites said he was straight, but the majority of guys on escort sites are gay or bisexual. He was tall, fair, reasonably good looking with a toned body, and he seemed to be on quite a lot of escort sites; I got the feeling he'd been around for a while.

I decided to email and see if he really was bi. I always imagine that bi men can't really be that into women's bodies – I don't know why I think that, especially as I'm a bi woman who loves men! I told him I was looking for him to meet with me and my boyfriend, and that I'd like a threesome, which would involve him giving my boyfriend oral sex. I was being very blunt, I know, but it was the only way I could find out if he was really bi. He said he wasn't into that sort of thing and wasn't what I was looking for, so I immediately wrote back and said that actually, he was exactly what I was looking for: a straight guy. It turned out he wasn't even aware that he'd been listed as being bi.

It would cost me £500 for him to travel to Nottingham and stay overnight. This seemed like a lot of money – that's a pair of Gucci shoes or a weekend away! I'd have been totally gutted if I'd spent all that money and not felt truly satisfied with my experience. It made me appreciate the gamble my clients take, especially those not that well-off, although they can read about other people's experiences with me, so they do have an idea what to expect from a date. I wondered how I would feel about paying for companionship; it would be weird to see the roles reversed – I'd be so nervous, and it would be odd to hand the envelope over and have the guy counting the money. I'd be totally out of my depth. For once I wouldn't feel in control, and that was a scary thought.

I'd want him to offer exactly what I don't – I'd want him to stay at mine, get a takeaway, and then spend the night making love. I wouldn't want him to do a 'me' and say we had to go out for dinner, or want to go to sleep at 12.30, or stick a snore strip on my nose, telling me not to disturb him in the night! Although I have to say, if I had him as a client, I would probably bend my usual strict rules and routine. In the end, I decided the experience wasn't really for me, so I didn't go for it.

CHAPTER 25:
It Ain't All Glamour...

I've had some embarrassing dates in my time. I once met a client at his home for a dinner date, and as I'd planned to drive home that night, I drove us to the restaurant. He directed me to a place in a small village, about five minutes away, which looked very nice from the outside. The food was lovely and we chatted away about our hobbies.

Suddenly I realised that my nose was dripping. He carried on talking and I was trying to sniffle away quietly, waiting for a break in the conversation to nip to the loo for some tissue. That break never came, so I had to interrupt, excuse myself and nip upstairs. When I sat back down to dinner, my stomach felt very bloated, like I really did need the loo. I was trying to keep focused on what he was saying, because I thought he might think I was a coke addict if I went to the loo again!

I attempted to take my mind off it, but my body had other ideas and I had to interrupt him again. This time, I made up a silly excuse about forgetting to go to the loo when I went to blow my nose, and got up from the table. Upstairs, it was very clear that something hadn't agreed with me. I could have stayed there for ages, but conscious of leaving him waiting I just hoped I'd be OK until I got back to my ex's house, where I was staying that evening to break up my journey.

When I went back to the table, I thanked him for the meal and we left the restaurant. As a hint, I mentioned that I had cramps in my tummy and when we got back to his place, I had to go again. I was terrified he would hear me as the bathroom was opposite his bedroom, and I was also worried about the smell. I was doubled over on the loo – it was horrible! I knew I'd have to go again, but I really wanted to be able to hold it off until I'd sorted him out. I was mortified when he went in the loo after me to brush his teeth, and I tried to look all sexy on the bed when he came out, but I just wanted to be home in bed. I knew he would have let me go, but I didn't want to disappoint him.

Somehow, I managed to hold off going to the loo while we played in bed. Almost as soon as I'd sorted him out, my cramps started again; I had to admit that I had a dodgy tummy and really wasn't well. I asked if I could shut the bedroom door while I went to the loo again. He thoughtfully fetched me an air freshener, but the whole episode was so embarrassing – I had never even met the guy before and I stank out his bathroom! I went back to the bedroom and hoped there would be no more. Though I was dreading the journey home, I snuggled up to him and we chatted. He said that even though I was poorly, he'd still had a lovely time and that he definitely wanted to see me again, and that next time it would be for an overnight. Sorted!

There's a lovely guy I've seen a few times who's 34, and he has learning difficulties. He's overweight and has a slight problem with B.O., and he wears glasses and has yellow teeth. He's a really sweet guy, but I have absolutely no idea where he gets his money from – as far as I know he only does voluntary work!

One night I accepted an overnight date with him. He wanted to take me to see Beyoncé in concert in Nottingham. He wore a smart suit with a tie – it looked totally out of place at the concert, bless him, but I did tell him he looked very smart! I arrived wearing tight jeans and boots, so we looked a bit odd together.

We ate in one of my favourite restaurants and then made our way to the concert nice and early; we were seated in the main area in front of the stage. There were some steps down to our seating area and Jack looked a bit uneasy, so I asked if I could help him. I took his water and was about to give him a shoulder to grab onto, when suddenly he pulled away and said, 'This is a bit embarrassing.' He proceeded to sit at the top of the stairs and bump down them on his bottom!

I tried hard not to giggle, because it did look quite comical. I wasn't aware he had any problems with stairs, so I just stood there bewildered, not quite sure what to do. Everyone turned around to watch him bumping down the stairs like a baby. Thankfully, after a few moments the staff noticed and two of them rushed to his aid. I felt a bit silly because if I'd known, I could have got help for him, but it all happened so quickly and he didn't even give me a chance. We were sitting about 20 rows back, but we did have a good view. He explained that there was something wrong with his feet, so he was unsteady on them. I expect most of the people there must have thought I was his carer, but he's very sweet and I genuinely enjoy our dates.

Age is not something that bothers me. In fact, give me a man in his sixties over a 30-year-old any day! They're generally more respectful, less demanding, and they want to please me too, so I didn't think I had an age limit. The biggest age gap I've had was when I was 26 and saw a doctor who was 69. However, a year or so ago I took a call from a well-spoken gentleman who sounded really elderly on the phone. He wanted to arrange just dinner, but he kept saying he was too old for me. I wasn't sure how old he was, and I didn't want to ask, so we arranged to meet for a two-hour lunch.

I arrived in the restaurant and saw this really old, but sweet-looking, overweight man hobbling towards me. It was him. He was lovely, and turned out to be one of the most interesting guys I've ever met, but he was in his early 90s! He had just written a book that had been published about his time in the Army during the war, and had brought a copy along with him. He spoke about the book and even had a photo of himself with Winston Churchill; he was so funny and had lots of interesting stories to tell – for once I didn't mind someone just talking about themselves, I was mesmerised listening to him. He said to me that he had never made love with a woman he hadn't been in love with, and then he said, 'I think I'm falling in love with you!' I found that highly amusing, so that's how he would justify sleeping with an escort. Bless him!

He asked whether he should book a hotel for our next meeting. I replied that although I thought he was a lovely guy, I wouldn't feel comfortable. I mean, what if he died on me? I know he would have died happy, but I would be horrified. Can you imagine explaining that one at the hotel? And think of the police calling his family! I don't think he would have been able to get it up anyway – he probably hadn't tried for a long time and just assumed he was still in working order. If he was, then good for him! I said I would be more than happy to book a date with him again and just have dinner, and that I would be happy to charge him a significantly lower rate, but I knew he probably wouldn't agree, and he hasn't contacted me since. I wonder if he ever found a lady to accommodate him.

One embarrassing time, when I wanted the ground to open up and swallow me whole, was when I met a lovely gentleman for an extended overnight date, which included a concert. It was a last-minute arrangement, but he was very sweet. We dined early at a pre-theatre dinner venue, and after a very tasty meal, we enjoyed the concert and retired to the hotel. As I've said before, I always look for signs that the gentleman is freshly showered, so when I went to the bathroom I was troubled to see no sign of an overnight bag. I brushed my teeth and felt irritated that he wouldn't bother to do the same; I tried to be tactful in the clumsy way that I am – I said I was nice and fresh, and had just brushed my teeth, then asked whether he'd like to brush his. When he said 'no', I was horrified, and I could feel myself losing patience. I asked him again, 'Don't you ever brush your teeth?' 'No,' he replied. I was furious and couldn't believe what I was hearing; I proceeded to rant about how disgusting he was.

He looked increasingly uncomfortable. 'I haven't got any teeth,' came the gummy reply. I was mortified. Me and my big mouth! We'd been out all evening – he'd even eaten steak – and I hadn't noticed. I have met old people previously who have had teeth, but they've not been visible when they speak and I assumed he was one of those. 'Oh,' I tried to say as casually and calmly as possible, 'why don't you get false ones?' He explained that he used to have them, but he was once out on a date and the teeth fell out onto his plate; ever since then, he didn't trust them to stay in! Which is understandable, I suppose. I tried to make it up to him in bed and give him a pleasurable time, but I still felt really silly. That was a memorable date – for all the wrong reasons!

CHAPTER 26:

What Now?

So, what do I want to do once my escorting career is over? I still lack confidence in my personal life, so maybe I'm not totally over the bullying I endured when I was younger; I always doubt myself and my decisions. I'm getting better, but I still have a long way to go.

People tell me I'd be good at counselling and friends appreciate the advice I give them. I love to help and advise people. I'd love to have an 'Agony Aunt' page in a magazine like *Cosmopolitan*, giving people relationship and sex advice based on the things I've learnt as an escort.

I went to see a counsellor myself for a few months because I was convinced there was something wrong with me, but he didn't think so, and I realised I was being far too hard on myself. I'm a perfectionist, which means that I focus on all my bad points and don't look at the good. I've still a way to go, but I'm getting there, and doing Aikido is improving my self-confidence.

I've always had a lot of empathy. It upsets me to see people upset, whether I know them or not. I don't read the newspapers or watch the news very often as I'll cry because I put myself in other people's shoes and imagine their pain and suffering. I also cry at films very easily, whether it's a sad or a romantic ending. Anything to do with romance makes me cry with happiness. I know, sad, isn't it? I love hearing stories from friends who are happy couples and I get especially emotional when I go to weddings; I suppose because I really want someone to love me that much and to want to marry me.

Being at work is an escape from my personal life, which can be full of ups and downs. I'm a worrier – I think too much about things and occasionally I let things get on top of me. I worry about time constantly: being late, or that I'm wasting time. At work I know exactly how I expect to be treated, and I'm confident with what I find acceptable and unacceptable.

When I was eight, I wanted to be a fashion designer. By the time I was 18, I knew it wasn't to be – I wasn't prepared to put the effort in at college. Sometimes I wonder if I suffered a mild form of Attention Deficit Disorder, not wanting to sit in a classroom and learn. If I could talk my way informally through a college course with no writing, I'd be a grade A student! Ever since I left my degree I've not known what I wanted to do with my life. Being very into fashion and good with people, I think I'd make a great personal shopper.

I envy people who are settled and happy in their careers. At various times in my life, I've spent hours trying to think what I'd like to do. I know I couldn't work in an office – I get bored easily and would need to do a job where there were challenges and some travel; I'd also have to work with people. Ideally, it would be my own company, one that's nothing to do with escorting, but what it might be, I haven't decided yet.

Many ladies get trapped in the world of escorting. They want to get out because they feel they've been doing it too long, but they're lost souls, not exactly sure how to move on. We get used to earning a certain amount of money, and then when we try to think what else we could do to bring in the same amount of capital with the same amount of flexibility, we come unstuck. What can you do without training or qualifications? I can't see me going back to being a student, but maybe I would, if only I had a clear idea what I wanted to do.

Some ladies with degrees and even higher qualifications still choose to escort. For some, it's the buzz of sleeping with different men, and the lifestyle that goes with it. Others maybe can't find a job even with their qualifications, so they start escorting while they look for work and they enjoy it so much that they carry on.

Those savvy enough save their money rather than squandering it on expensive handbags and shoes, and either set up their own businesses or buy into property or shares. I'm sorry to say that I've never really saved much money, which I regret now, but I do have my own property so I have something to show for all my hard work. I'm very careful with my money now, but there's not so much work around as there was years ago. The market is becoming saturated. More and more ladies are turning to escorting, so there's more choice, and there has been a steady rise in the number of ladies from Eastern Europe coming to the UK, many of whom are undercutting the standard UK rates, so men expect more and want to pay less.

Escorting becomes a way of life, and it's all I've known. I haven't had a 'proper' job for ten years, and I've worked for myself for nine years now. I don't know if I could work for someone else, because I'm so used to doing things my way and working when I want. What kind of job can I do? I'm always told that I'd be a good PA and that I'm good with people. Even so, how many people would offer me a job if they saw 'high-class escort for eight years' on my CV? How many would look at the positive qualities that I need to have for escorting? Empathy, an ability to mix and communicate with people in all levels of society and to make people feel comfortable quickly, they're all skills I need in my work. I'm a good organiser and have to be disciplined. Also, I'm a good listener and a good talker, but would people see past the 'escort'? Somehow I doubt it!

Eventually I'd love to build my confidence up enough to try being a presenter on TV. I don't take myself too seriously, and most of my friends think I'd be really good at it. I'd like to do something like *Street Date* – a project that involves getting out and about, interacting with different people on a mission, rather than standing in front of a big audience. That would terrify me! Being interested in people and psychology I am a massive reality T.V fan, so maybe I could do a reality show, and try and train up a 'wannabe' escort from a bunch of hopefuls? Or be like a *Supernanny* for relationships, visiting couples at home to help them sort out their problems? Perhaps I'll do a fly on the wall documentary showing how I integrate back into 'normal' society. One thing I am gutted to be missing out on is the chance to be on Richard and Judy's book club promoting my book! I've been a big fan of theirs, and was so disappointed when they stopped their show.

I'm keen to start a new chapter in my life and who knows where this book will take me? I'd love to be successful at another business before having children. As I'm one of four, I'd like a big family, and I'm conscious of my biological clock ticking! I've made some wonderful friends and had some amazing experiences, but I'm 33 now, and it's time to sort my life out!

Any suggestions or job offers, please email me! b@miss-b.net

CHAPTER 27:

Thoughts from Friends and Family

Sensei Ken

Beki walked into my office in Jan 2006. Her appointment was to last for about an hour, after which she would be invited to make a potentially life-changing decision.

My name is Ken, or Sensei as many people call me. I am a professional Martial Arts teacher, and I own a full-time school in Nottingham that teaches Aikido. A Japanese martial art, which although often described as non-violent, Aikido is the choice of military and police forces worldwide as a system of personal safety. The main focus of my school is life skills and personal safety and awareness. I have over 340 students from all ages and all walks of life.

This confident, pretty young blonde girl didn't quite fit the mould of most of the people who cross my threshold to embark on the way of the warrior. The path to Black Belt is a path fraught with trial and hardship, often literally a journey of blood, sweat and tears, and in my school if you start, I want to see you finish. Sadly, many fall before they complete this first step to Black Belt.

I never judge a book by its cover, but it's human nature to make a few assessments on first meetings. Looking at the long, manicured nails I couldn't help but wonder if this slight young lady would have what it takes. Still, if she was up for it, then as her teacher, I would do whatever it takes to get her there. As a routine part of the induction interview, I asked her what she did for a living. 'I run my own business,' she replied. I was impressed, not an easy thing to do, especially for someone so young. So naturally, I asked her what the nature of her business was. Without hesitation, and totally unperturbed, she replied that she was an escort.

Being a martial artist for over 30 years, and having spent 22 years in the military travelling the world, I have seen a few things and have been in a few interesting situations, so it's not often I am stopped in my tracks, but Beki did just that, albeit for just a moment, but it seemed like way too long for me. I certainly didn't want her to think me rude, so I quickly mustered a response. The thing that caused me to pause a second was not what she did, but how confidently she told me. I was impressed for the second time. I think my reply to her statement was, 'Wow, that's cool, how interesting.' Then I thought, 'Well good for you!' She asked me not to tell anyone else in the school as some people may think less of her because of it. I was pleased that clearly she trusted me, and offered that trust for, as yet, nothing in return. Maybe she could do this Aikido thing, after all.

I was a little surprised when she told me that the self-defence skills we teach here was not the drive behind her walking through the door – rather, she wanted confidence. Now I felt a little confused. I don't know too much about the escort profession, but I would have thought personal safety was essential and she didn't look like she needed confidence. It turned out Beki knew exactly what she was looking for.

Beki has been with me for over two and a half years now and has her second Kyu belt. Her Black Belt test should happen in about 18 months or so. If she tests on time, it will have taken her four years or so to get to Black Belt, which is about average. For those that can go the distance, that is – many don't make it even to Brown Belt. She has been both one of my best students and also one of my most challenging. Out of the 'blood, sweat and tears' thing, the tears are winning hands-down. It's been a challenge for me to coach Beki to where I need her to be; to change her thinking and to find the fighter in this girly girl. But the fighter is there. Beki just doesn't quit, she just keeps going in spite of the frustration she often feels. The one-on-one coaching sessions in my office – just Beki, me and a box of tissues – are becoming rare. She is growing, and becoming stronger and more confident all the time. Sometimes it's two steps forward, one step back, but we are moving forward, that's the main thing. The future is never certain and we have a way to go yet, but I think she has got what it takes. She has needed help, but in the end she has shown the courage and determination to get this far. I think she will make it to Black Belt, and beyond.

I have absolutely no issue at all with Beki's chosen profession. Over the years, my partner and I have established a friendship with Beki outside the dojo. She is a warm and friendly person, intelligent and honest, and is giving her training everything she has. What more could you ask of someone? Like any of my students, I would do anything to help her in time of need, or if called upon to do so. Your profession, doctor, lawyer, escort, builder, etc. has no bearing at all in my book. Who you are is what is important to me.

Pete, my brother

I don't remember you telling me you were going to work as an escort – you sort of drifted into it. I do, however, remember thinking it was a good way to get some quick money, get on the property ladder, and get some finance for the next step – whatever that might have been. I think escorting is similar to prostitution, and that some clients may see it as a more acceptable form of prostitution with less risk. Obviously, though, you choose the clients you want. You have led a very different life and are used to a very different lifestyle to the rest of us, which can alienate both you and the rest of the family, but I'm not really embarrassed about your job. I tell people what you do, but I don't go any further into it. I'm not sure how years of escorting will affect any future career or prepare you for anything else; I didn't expect what I thought was a quick way for you to earn some good money to turn into such a lengthy 'career'.

I think you have been used to the lifestyle for so long that it is what you expect now, and that will not change. Seeing as you went into it at such an early age, it's really all I've known you as and I have no doubt that it has affected you as a person, but who knows what you would be like, had you done something different with your life? Maybe better, maybe worse – we'll never know. I think the rest of the family share similar views to me, but you are my sister and I love you for better, for worse.

My friend and ex-boyfriend Keith

I've known Bec since I was 16, and she was 15. I remember the first time I saw her in Matlock Park – she caught my eye as she was wearing Levis that were ripped across both bum cheeks, exposing her bum. She certainly stood out from the crowd and I remember thinking, wow! I couldn't believe my luck when I found out she fancied me.

We went out with each other initially for three months, but saw each other on and off for about four years. I soon realised that she was mature far beyond her years. She seemed to know what she wanted, and how to get it. She wasn't your stereotypical clueless 15-year-old girl, she was very much one of the lads. I remember watching porn with my mates and their girlfriends would be there, as was Bec. All the girls would make a real fuss about the porn, and Bec would always love watching it. I thought she seemed sexually and emotionally advanced beyond her years.

I remember long pauses in our casual relationship as she was away at college and university for three years, and when she was home she was often up and down the country, going to various raves and parties. She was always very sociable and loved meeting new people.

I hadn't been in touch with her for a while as she started a long-term relationship with James. I heard on the grapevine they were no longer going out, so I rang her out of the blue as I was curious what adventures she had been up to. I asked her where she was. She told me she was at Derby station and she seemed a little apprehensive as she paused and said she wasn't sure if I'd want to be friends with her anymore once she confessed where she was going – which was on an escort job. My initial thought was that I wasn't surprised as she'd always been a bit wild, but I did feel a twinge of jealousy and was concerned for her safety as she confessed she hadn't seen the guy she was meeting before. It didn't change my opinion of her and I knew I still wanted us to be friends.

We occasionally met up for a drink in a local pub, and sometimes I'd be with my mate and we'd both laugh at the funny stores she told us about her escorting jobs. She's had boyfriends since she's been escorting and although I didn't see her much, we've always maintained our friendship. Presently we catch up about once a month for dinner, and speak about once a week. We both chew each other's ears off and support each other.

She's been an escort now for eight years and I've known her over half my life. She's one of the most grounded people I know, and to me she hasn't changed as a person. I wish her the best of luck and long may our friendship continue!

Katie G, Matlock friend

I'd always known of Beki, as she was someone who certainly stood out in the crowd – I think the first time I saw her was in Harvey's in Matlock and she was in some crazy rubber hot pants outfit and pigtails in her hair – I remember some of the other girls were turning their noses up but I was secretly quite jealous that I couldn't get away with outfits like that! I also know Beki used to get bullied – some of the lads I hung around with used to slag her off and call her horrible names. However I never listened to any of this, and certainly never judged Beki when, through the Matlock grapevine, I would hear gossip and rumours about her and what she was doing with her life.

The first time I properly met Beki, many years later, we hit it off straight away, especially after I told her I was moving to Nottingham. We swapped numbers and agreed to meet up some time. Our friendship went from there and was assisted by our mutual love of Sunday afternoon wine and cocktails in the bars of Nottingham!

When I met Beki, I was fully aware of what she did for a living, and was intrigued to find out more about her and what she does. Beki is very open about her work, so it didn't take long for me to hear all the juicy details. I don't have any problem with what she does, she is professional in what she does and more importantly she is intelligent and would never do a job that sounded dodgy or that she didn't feel 100% happy with.

Beki is an amazingly great person to be around as her personality is bubbly, friendly and warm. I think this is what makes her so good at what she does. When you are with her, she gives you her 100% attention and is always genuinely interested in what you have to say. Often when we are out having dinner and a good old chat, I catch myself thinking – wow, some people have to pay for Beki's fun company, and I get it all for free!

I can't imagine many other people being able to do what

Beki does so well, she runs a tight ship, is very organised and works very hard especially with her web marketing – a side of things that I don't think too many people think about.

I am proud to be Beki's friend.

Aunty Sue

The first time I met Beki she was about 7 years of age. She was always a lively child. I am her aunt, married to her mother's youngest brother. From the very beginning Beki and I always had a special bond. We seemed to 'hit it off' even when she was very young. I don't think I knew why in the early years but I do believe that we both feel we are different from our siblings. We are both interested in fashion and like having nice things around us.

I recall when she was about 8 years of age trying to put some make up on her. She ended up looking like a clown – we both thought it was very funny. Even at that age we had a bond.

When we first met I had no children of my own, so my husband's nieces and nephews were the next best thing. We used to see the children quite often so we got to know them well.

I remember very vividly the first time Beki told me she was going to become an escort. We were in a café not far from where she was living at her mum and dad's. She was looking for a phone for her new job. I asked her what her new job was all about and she said that men would take her out for dinner at their expense, and that she would be paid to spend time with them. I remember pondering if that meant she had to sleep with them. I am not naïve and perhaps I was somewhat in denial but I did not ask the question and it was not discussed at that time. My daughter Vickie, who was present, was only thirteen years of age so I thought it inappropriate to discuss. I did think she would be sleeping with them and I was not shocked knowing that her previous job had been a lap dancer.

It was some time before we discussed her job in more detail. It was at a family gathering after a few drinks. Beki confirmed that she did have sex on her escort dates.

Beki being an escort has never affected our relationship. She is still the same person. If I were to be asked the question 'would you rather she did something else?' my answer would be yes. But if what she is doing makes her happy then it's her choice. If asked how I would feel if my daughter wanted to escort - naturally I would not like it. However Beki is not hurting anyone and some would say that she is offering a service to help some people, and that she plays a part in keeping some marriages together.

I do have concerns about her future when age becomes the better of her – what will she do in the future? After saying that, I know that Beki is resourceful so hopefully something will come along. Whatever happens I know that we will remain good friends and I love her for the person she is.

Vickie, my cousin

I can remember when Beki told me about her career move. We were in Matlock and she received a phone call from a friend. She told me that he was helping her set up a website, so I asked her what it was for. I can't remember exactly how she explained it to me as I was about 13 at the time, but I can remember thinking, oh, OK, as if she was telling me, 'I'm just popping out to the shops...' It certainly didn't change our relationship or my opinion of my cousin, I think maybe because she was older than me and I really looked up to her, but also because we were, and still are, close. Family gatherings were always the same; I don't recall anyone acting any differently towards Beki.

As I grew older and understood more, I had a look at her website. I can remember being quite intrigued and asking her questions about the type of clients she would see, where she would go, what she would do. Some of it was very glamorous: she would get taken on lovely holidays, stay in beautiful hotels, she always had very nice clothes, shoes and handbags bought for her.

I guess the only thing I wonder about now is what job will she do next? How will she be perceived by potential employers? They will be looking through CVs and come to 'Rebecca Dakin' – what will they do, screw up the CV and not give her a chance? Because I know her, I know she is not the stereotype people may think of when they think of escorting, like Leanne Battersby in *Corrie* and how people looked down their noses at her. Will this image that's portrayed hinder her?

My friend JZ

I met Beki about a year ago, through a mutual friend, out in a bar in town. We had all met up for a few drinks, and then a few of us, including Beki, went on from there to some other bars to go dancing or whatever. Thinking back, my initial impression was that she looked really good – I liked her hair and style – and that she seemed friendly, fun and quite sweet.

Although I hadn't even wondered what she did for a living, someone already told me she was an escort by the time she mentioned it to me that evening. My initial reaction in my mind was pretty much, 'Ah, that kind of makes sense' as she had a look that fitted the discreet upmarket escort image: big boobs, slim legs, perfect make-up, elegant but glam clothes and shoes, sexy hair. Not tacky or too much flesh out, but pretty much immaculate and well groomed. I hadn't glammed myself up that night and Beki was the kind of girl you might not want to stand next to, if she's done up and you're not, but there's something in her manner that made me think, you're safe, you are, it's good to have met you, rather than feel threatened or insecure.

When she told me herself, as part of a wider conversation, what her profession was, I just said something like, 'Ah, right', and our chitchat continued as normal. I was aware some people might be a bit gossipy about her work, so I didn't mention that someone had taken it on themselves to tell me. It wasn't something that even mildly surprised or shocked me, or altered my perception of her in any way. For a start, I'd only just met her, and whatever people choose to do is OK with me, I'm not someone to judge people or be disapproving. Beki seemed cool and genuine, and we just got on and kept in touch from then on.

As me and Beki got to know each other, my initial assessment of her was about right – she's a great mate, considerate, fun and interesting to talk to, and we just easily became friends. Over time, I've also come to see the insecurities and contradictions in her character. Everyone has these, but from what I've seen so far, I think that Beki's are very much linked to self-image and being desired on a physical level, and I do think this has influenced the choices she has made along the way to do with her career. I do sometimes find her principles odd or funny, or a contradiction to what she does for a living, but I understand she has managed to maintain a lot of her balance, self-respect and professionalism through this attitude, which could otherwise be easily lost or undermined through doing the work she does.

As for how it affects our friendship, it doesn't. It's just what she does to pay her bills, although I suppose it has more potential to provide the topic of discussion for a girls' night in than my own graft does. It's always interesting to hear about her latest job: she's got these lovely tales of fantastic restaurants and hotels she's visited, and then some cringe-worthy stories. I don't know how she does it when I hear about some of the clients; even just having to go for dinner and engage in conversation with some of these men would be too much for me.

Every now and then I do have to check myself to not be jealous of some of the bonuses of her job – 5-star hotels, jewellery, designer shopping trips and expensive cosmetics to help her look even better, all that kind of thing, but I know it's not for me, so fair play and good luck to her. I bet plenty of girls disrespect or begrudge her, or see her as a threat, or become suspicious of her motives around men, or experience a whole range of issues, but these are results of their own insecurities about themselves and their relationships. I don't have that so there's no problems like that between me and Beki; she's just my mate who's doing what she does.

I'm glad for Beki that she's writing this book, even if she has to burn certain bridges behind her, if it goes to print; I think it's important she opens up the options for her future. The whole process of learning about writing and publishing is a new challenge and experience away from the escorting business, and that's good news for her confidence and self-esteem. I believe Beki has loads of skills that she could apply to other careers. After all, she has been running and managing her own successful business for years now.

As for men and love – that's the hardest one for me to decide how I feel about it. I can't imagine there are many men out there who could really be unaffected by her work, if they were in a serious relationship with her. And I know Beki wants love, a man and a family in the future. I don't think that can happen with the right kind of bloke while she still works as an escort, which is another reason why it's good for her to be looking at moving out of that industry. And then she'll need a really confident, secure man, who doesn't get threatened by her past, and who can show her he loves her for who she is, and give her all the reassurance and attention that she needs.

Best of luck to her with the book and any opportunities it may throw up for her – I admire her motivation and focus, and I believe she deserves to continue to be successful in her life.

My friend, Daniel James

I first met Hazel Bazel (as I call her) when my ex-boyfriend and I were travelling around Australia in 2005. We all joined a coach tour that was picking us up from Sydney and taking us up the east coast of Oz. On the first morning, before anyone knew each other, we had to stand at the front of the coach and talk a bit about ourselves. I just remember Beki coming to the front of the coach and being so hungover that she could barely talk. She sat down before she had finished what she was saying and rested her head on the tour rep's shoulder.

From this first meeting I made a few assumptions, firstly that she was about ten years younger than she actually is, that she was just like any other normal traveller and that she knew the tour rep. Turns out, I was wrong on every assumption!

As the tour went on, my ex and I became really good friends with Beki, and along with a couple of others, formed quite a tight little group. We obviously found out about what she did for a living as time went on, and I can honestly say it didn't change my opinion of her one bit. She has the warmest character that you are naturally drawn to and makes everyone feel like she has known them for years – hence my assumption about the tour rep.

I think it was Beki's openness and honesty that made it so easy to accept what she did for a living as if she had said she was a doctor or a lawyer. Even when Beki wasn't in the group, nobody felt the need to talk about her behind her back, really because there was nothing to say that you couldn't ask to her face.

In the situation in which we met, you get to know people really quickly and forge quite strong friendships as we were living in each other's pockets for three weeks. At the end of the tour we vowed to stay in touch, which I am happy to say we have. We speak on the phone at least once a month and it is never a short chat – I need to make sure I have at least an hour free! Beki asks me questions about my job, and I ask her questions about hers.

I don't know if my being gay has anything to do with the fact that I am more open to somebody else's sexuality or how they use it, but I do know that all of my friends that have been introduced to her say what a lovely person she is.

My brother Andy

I was shocked and disappointed when you first told me you were going to be an escort, and I remember thinking there's got to be other jobs, and I'd rather you did something else. I knew what escorting involved, and my view is that it's upmarket prostitution. I guess there's a difference between escorting and prostitution: as an escort you have to be able to present yourself well and be more adaptable socially than a prostitute.

I know that the job has given you some amazing opportunities. It's well paid, and you've been to a lot of places, different countries and cities, fine dining and grand hotels, but at the same time, at what cost? Sometimes I feel like you're degrading yourself. I don't want to hear or talk about your work. In fact, the more I know, the more I dislike what you're doing. Ignorance makes it easier to deal with. People know I don't like talking about it, so no one mentions it or asks me.

From my point of view, you've had opportunities, done a lot and seen a lot, but it will be a happy day when you finish escorting. When this book is published even though more people will know what you've done, at least if anyone asks me I can say you're no longer doing it. I don't know if you're now too old, but one job where you get to travel and use the same skills looking after customers and see the world would be an air hostess, but really, I would just rather you did anything other than what you're doing now.

I will be pleased and happier when you do something else. I don't think it affects our relationship, but there's a big part of your life at the moment that I have no interest in.

Andrea, solicitor and lecturer

I've known Beki for around five years. She was our neighbour for a number of years, and I got to know her gradually during that time. Quite a few residents of the complex where we all lived were intrigued by Beki before any of us had even spoken to her – this was because someone had started a rumour that she was a porn star! To add fuel to the fire, they'd seen a huge waterbed being delivered, so gossip was rife.

Beki also stood out as she always looked so glamorous when she was heading out, so she certainly turned a few heads, and naturally, the men in the complex would brag that their neighbour was a porn star and wonder what went on in her apartment!

It was on a night out with all the neighbours, and after a few drinks, when I plucked up the courage to ask what Beki did and I was really impressed by her open, honest answers to the barrage of questions that followed from everyone else ('Do your parents know?' 'How did you get into it?' 'Do your clients visit your apartment?' 'So, does that mean you have to sleep with your clients then?' 'What are they like?' 'How much do you charge?') It was quite fascinating as none of us had ever met a real-life escort before.

Despite being a world away from what I do, and still completely intriguing, I don't think Beki's profession had any negative impact on our friendship – Beki is a fun, kind and thoughtful friend, she just has more interesting work stories than I do!

My Aunty Kate

I have known you since I got together with your Uncle Will, so that would be about 30 years! I found out what you did for a living when you told me about eight years ago. When you initially told me I was quite amused, actually. I certainly wasn't shocked, for some reason, but if you had been my daughter, I would probably have felt differently. You would think that someone doing your job would change fundamentally in some way, but you have always stayed the same. You don't try and flash your money around, or try to outdo your brothers and sister materialistically, or your cousins. We don't hear you bragging about what you've got, but neither are you ashamed about what you have achieved. You remain in some ways unworldly, which only adds to your normality. You haven't gone off the rails either, which is to your credit as I expect you have mixed with some rather colourful characters on occasions!

You seemed to conduct your business in a rather tactful way and I always thought you made it appear very normal and nothing to fuss about! Because you treated it like that in our company, I guess we just accepted it like that.

I don't think you have gone down in anyone's estimation within the family, saving maybe your grandparents. Because of the era that they were brought up in, they would have found the situation difficult, not least because of their love for you. One always wants the best for those you love, so those closest to you would have found it very difficult to accept initially. Even in this modern world we live in, old-fashioned values still hold true.

We would love you to meet someone, fall in love and live happily ever after with a lovely man, but the trouble is a lovely man probably wouldn't want you with your history, and so I think we all worry that ultimately you will lose out in some way. Emotional enrichment is a very satisfying and uplifting state to find oneself in and I feel sad that you may never experience it now.

You come from a very stable and loving family background and I think it is to their credit too that you have remained so normal. They never shut you out when they found out about your job, and from what I have observed, they have always been there as a safety net for you whenever you have needed it. You have a very good relationship with them all and I know you have treated your mother a lot, which I think is lovely of you.

Jenny

I first met Beki at the Aikido Christmas night out in 2006; we ended up sitting opposite each other. Although I was not near the people I knew from my classes, we had a good laugh. Aikido nights out are always a bit wild as there is a certain level of trust already established – just lots of drinking and having a laugh. We ended up in Oceana and all the girls were dancing. The girls I was friendlier with decided to leave for another party – Beki persuaded me to stay out with her and I was definitely not ready to go home just yet!

We had a great time, dancing the night away and having a good laugh. It later turned out that this was the night she told some of the girls what she did for a living. I must have been somewhere else at the time, as this is something I would not have forgotten!! I didn't see Beki for a while after that night. It was a few months later, on another Aikido night out, when we got talking again and we got on really well. I asked her what she did for a living as part of general conversation. She mumbled something back, and I got the feeling she did not want to tell me, so left it there.

I was given a lift home by another friend, and asked her if she knew what Beki did for a living, because something was bugging me – she was beautiful and glamorous, always dressed immaculately. And being a girl with an eye for beautiful things such as shoes, jewellery and handbags, I had to ask. Although this all sounds very superficial, I already knew she was such a great person! We swapped numbers that night and we have become increasing close ever since.

When I confessed to knowing what Beki did, she thought I already knew. We have clicked as friends and I love her being in my life for who she is – a fabulous person and a great friend; we share some similar feelings derived from things that have happened in our lives such as childhood bullying, boys/men not finding us attractive (when now we're actually probably some of the best looking girls around, not to blow our own trumpets!). I find her professional life interesting as it is the opposite of what I do – Human Resources and Payroll – and is something I had not much idea about before I met Beki. I've learned a lot from Beki on a personal level; she has helped me through various difficulties in my life recently, and I am so grateful for that. Beki is one of the most special and giving people I know and I look forward to many more memorable times in our, hopefully, long future as friends!

Nat

I first met Beki when I was 15. She knew a friend of mine and we were going into Matlock one morning and Beki (at that time, 17) and a mate of hers had been out raving and were sat on a bench looking very cool and chilled out, and tired.

We said hello, and that was about it. We first met properly when I was 16, and I was on my lunch break from work, sat alone in the park, and I think Beki was doing the same. We started talking, and the main topic was how much we loved going out, and started talking about Chesterfield on a Thursday night; we made loose plans to arrange to go together some time. Beki came into the pharmacy where I worked later that day and said, 'Fancy going tonight?' Which we did. I remember being sat in the bus on the back seat and we just talked and laughed, and it was as if I'd known her for ages. I'm fairly sure I'm not the only person to think this.

This ability to get on with people is one of the reasons she is a good escort, in my opinion. We became very good friends and shared a love of dancing, hardcore, boys and generally having a laugh. It was Beki, being two years older than me, who first took me to the Doncaster Warehouse, which was one of the coolest underground clubs back in the day. We have been clubbing all over, including Derby, Nottingham, Manchester, Leicester, Sheffield, and we always had an amazing time.

When Beki first told me she had been working as an escort

I wasn't shocked as she had always been pretty wild. I was intrigued and wanted to know more, of course, and I also found it a bit funny, and maybe I was a bit envious... thinking 'Oh my God, you're earning HOW MUCH MONEY?!' As we have been good friends for a long time, I have heard all about the good and the bad and the ugly, and devour the details with relish. I suppose now it's been a good few years, I probably ask less and less, and will have the normal conversation like, 'How's work?' etc., but not go into detail. It's just a job, after all! Well, that's how I see it now.

Has it changed her? Well, I would say she is now more assertive and particular. That may come with getting older as we all develop better ideas of what we want and don't want.

I don't think it's affected her self-image or confidence at all. In fact, I think if anything, she is probably more confident. The only way it affects our friendship is if we make arrangements and it's made clear that they could be cancelled due to work, which can be disheartening at first, but actually it's never happened so it's not affected anything at all so far.

This is one of the world's oldest professions and why not? If it doesn't affect a person in a negative way, I do not see the problem. I will add that the way Beki runs her business is impeccable and I know that she wouldn't put herself in any danger.... I do realise the other end of the scale can be a whole lot darker, however.

Mum

Rebecca was always a bit of a rebel in her early teenage years; she had a focused determination to fulfil dreams that for most young girls are just dreams. As parents you can have certain control over your children and hope to instil discipline through love and care; however, as they begin to grow up, this can become more difficult. You cannot lock a child away from the world they are to grow up in – all you can try and achieve, by being open and honest, is for them to learn the difference between right and wrong, how to behave in society and to instil a sense of responsibility, confidence and pride in themselves. You hope that they will use their talents to forge a path towards a successful career in which they will be happy, fulfilled and contented.

Rebecca had, and still has, such creative talent – but when she decided (and was determined!) to go dancing instead of finishing her university degree, I was concerned at the route she seemed to be taking. I suppose it came as no real surprise, after a very naïve beginning on that route, she ended up working as an escort. I was saddened by her choice of career (if that's what you call it?) – I felt she was worthy of something better; something that did not mean she was selling herself. I did feel some relief when she made it clear (after investigating all the options of escorting) that she knew the clientele she was hoping to attract and that she would always leave the details of her work with us. I think my main concern was her safety; in that line of work, there must be an element of risk.

I cannot say that I was happy with her choice of career – I felt her artistic talent, her organisational skills and her charm could have led elsewhere. However, we all make our own choices in life, and maybe any other choice she might have considered would not have given her so many diverse, exciting and adventurous experiences.

CHAPTER 28

Top Tips for GFF Escorts

Top Tips for GFE Escorts

To be a good GFE escort you need to be:

Attentive and a good listener

Giving your date your full attention is extremely important. They need to feel that you are interested and focused on them. I know of ladies who are constantly glancing around to see who is looking at them, watching to see how many admiring looks they get. I just think that's rude. I treat people with the same respect I would like myself. My eyes are focused on the gentleman I am with. I listen, ask questions and generally show an interest in them.

A good talker

Many men are very shy, especially with someone attractive. You need to be able to lead the conversation and avoid it drying up. There should be no awkward silences. Basic conversation starters for me include, first how their day has been, what they do for a living, how far they have travelled. If anything has happened to me during my journey I always find this to be a good icebreaker when I arrive. It might be that I got totally lost trying to find them in the hotel and had to walk past Reception a few times and received some dubious looks from the staff! If the hotel is large and I have to walk down a labyrinth of corridors to get there, I usually make a joke, like, 'I see they've put you out of the way, you must have looked like trouble!' If there's no peephole on the door, I usually acknowledge that too, saying they weren't able to peep to see if it was me! Really, I say anything to break the ice as quickly as possible when I enter the room.

Other conversation points include music, the weather, holidays, education, world issues, travel, hobbies, food, wine, art.

The number one topic to avoid is family. If the guy is married he may not want to be reminded of that. If he talks about his family, fine, just don't ask. I talk about my family, but I wouldn't tell them if I had a partner or children because I want them to feel that I am single. For me it's all part of the fantasy. If it was obvious I had had children then I wouldn't deny it, if I was asked, but I wouldn't mention my partner if I had one. Other topics to avoid are religion and politics and other dates you have been on or are about to go on. The gentleman does not want to be reminded that you are not exclusively his, even if he is married!

Able to put people at ease, and bring them out of their shell

Some guys are so nervous they are shaking when I arrive. It's up to me to make them feel comfortable as quickly as possible, and I usually do this by leading the conversation, so they don't have to think. It's no good just talking about yourself: you need to show an interest in them and ask questions. You also need to read their body language, and try and work out how they are feeling. If someone is really nervous, it's always best to try a bit of humour. If you can make them laugh, it's definitely a good ice-breaker. Afterwards, follow it up with light-hearted conversation.

A sexual, affectionate and tactile person

In my opinion you cannot offer a Girlfriend Experience if you don't kiss. If you don't want to kiss, that's your prerogative, but I don't think you should advertise yourself as a GFE. Not kissing is interpreted as detaching yourself from the experience.

What surprises me is that the thing most men seem to be missing at home is affection. It really isn't just about the sex. I always thought it was just women that wanted this, but this profession has made me see otherwise. I am very affectionate and tactile; I love stroking and kissing, however I don't like public displays of affection, and that's not just for escorting, it's also for my personal life, so I wouldn't let any of my dates grope me or constantly kiss me in public. I don't mind the odd peck, but definitely no tongues until the bedroom!

Once in the bedroom, I like to take my time and set the scene with candles and music. I like lots of slow foreplay and massage, and plenty of kissing. After we have had our fun, I usually just stroke the guy and cuddle until it's time to leave, or go to sleep.

Comfortable and confident with your body, whatever your size

There's nothing more attractive for a guy than a woman who is comfortable with her size and body. Contrary to what you may believe, you don't have to be a stick-thin, big-chested Scandinavian blonde to make money as an escort. Some men like big women, some like skinny, others like a small chest, others larger chests, some like blondes and some prefer redheads. The only thing you have to be is confident. They don't want to see a lady who insists on having the lights out and diving under the covers (that's often what they get at home!), because men love visuals.

Intelligent with common sense

When I say 'intelligent', I don't mean you need a degree or A-levels, as I have neither of these. I mean, able to hold an intelligent conversation.

Reliable

Really, it goes without saying: if you want to be successful, you need to be reliable. It's no good arranging a date and then deciding you don't feel like going.

I can count on my fingers the number of cancellations I have made in my eight-year career. That, on average, is less than two a year. If you are genuinely ill or have a proper excuse, then you need to let the guy know as soon as possible. Maybe offer him a discount or something for next time to compensate for the inconvenience. You don't want word to get round that you're unreliable or this will cost you future bookings.

I heard about a guy recently who arranged a date and had gone out of his way to rearrange his diary to accommodate the lady he was due to see. He checked into the hotel. She called to say she was held up in traffic and he rearranged his meetings so he could still see her. He then called her back, and she said it was too late and she had already set off home. Shocking! Needless to say, he wasn't a happy bunny.

A good organiser

A diary or Filofax is a must and you need to set your own way of doing things: you can get a whole diary full of dates that never happen, and you may have turned work down. I don't confirm anything without a booking reference for a hotel, and I also take a full name, and contact telephone number. If someone wants me to put something in my diary and then they'll call a few days before to confirm, I say that I can't keep the date free for them until I have the details I need. If they think their plans might change, I ask them to call back when they know for sure if they can make it. Hopefully I'll still be available. Some guys forget that although they are arranging to see escorts in their free time, it's not the escort's free time, it's our work time.

If you can't make a date and you have a booking for that evening, then it's a good idea to ask the guy if he would like you to contact him if your diary changes. It does happen, unfortunately.

If a guy cancels because of work it's likely he has a job where his plans can change at short notice, so the same thing could happen again. If I get a cancellation for whatever reason, I say I need to take a deposit to rearrange another date to prove they are not a timewaster. If they cancel again, they don't get their money back because it may have cost me work.

You don't need to mention other dates. If you're unavailable for a few weeks and clients comment about you being busy, it's good to remind them that you do have a social life and that you're very selective and only see a few dates. Because if you can't make a date for a good few weeks, they may assume you are working every night!

Hygienic

You might think this goes without saying. Well, so it should! Clean, fresh underwear and clothes are essential. I shower and pamper myself before I set off for my date, but if I don't feel fresh when I arrive, I shower again.

I use panty liners to keep my underwear looking fresh, but obviously I remove them before I get intimate. Also, I smother myself in scented body lotion and keep myself trimmed in all the right places. I also get regular check-ups at the GU clinic – I go once every three months. I'd advise any escort to do the same, and to let the clinic know that they are an escort – the nurses can't properly advise on safe sex if they don't know the full story.

Punctual

I'm one of those people who really cares about being on time: I get very stressed and distressed if I'm late or think I might be late. Even if I'm going to be five minutes late, I call, and when I arrive, I apologise profusely. I once got the time wrong and got in my car at 7p.m. before realising my date was due to start then! As soon as I realised, I panicked. I debated whether to call him (it was before the days of hands-free), and be even later, or just to get there and then explain.

I decided, as I would only be 10–15 minutes late, I would explain when I arrived. By that time, I was extremely flustered and apologetic. The guy had never seen an escort before and soon forgot about being nervous because of the flap I was in! He said it really broke the ice, and he was touched that I had got myself so stressed about it, because he could tell that I really cared. Seven years down the line, I still meet him for dates.

All the time, I hear shocking stories of ladies not turning up, or waltzing in two hours late, without even an apology or explanation. In some cases, they don't show at all!

Well-mannered

Good manners go a long way. It's true what they say; always remember your Ps and Qs. You need to be able to go to a top restaurant and have good table manners. Basic things count, like not speaking with your mouth full. Not being greedy, or having too much to drink. You need to know which cutlery to use for each course. Also, you need to know the correct etiquette.

There are many good books and websites to help you with this. A few basic table manners are:

1 Sit up straight
2 Don't speak with a mouth full of food
3 Chew quietly and try not to slurp

4 Keep bites of food small
5 Eat at a leisurely pace
6 Don't wave utensils in the air
7 Keep your elbows off the table
8 Don't reach across the table
9 Don't forget to say please and thank you
10 Always excuse yourself when leaving the table

Well-presented and take pride in your appearance

For every date, I make sure that I turn up looking my best. I am always freshly shaven, showered and tidy, and I make sure my nails are filed and looking nice, toenails trimmed. I don't wear polish often because it chips too quickly and I would never go on a date with chipped polish. My clothes are clean, fresh and well-pressed. I also ask what the gentleman is wearing, so I can dress accordingly.

Adaptable to situations and different people

Generally, I find I can get on with most people. If you have this quality, it will be extremely useful in your career as an escort. One day you might be with a high-flying businessman the next you could meet someone who stacks shelves in a local supermarket! You need to be comfortable around people and able to adapt to different situations and personalities. There are guys who meet escorts because they lack social skills, and an escort has to be able to put people like that at ease.

Diplomatic

As an escort you really must try and think before you speak, which I sometimes find difficult – I am a very outspoken person. I have had guys boast to me about how they are deceiving their wives, and in that situation I find it very difficult to keep quiet. I mean, what can I say? I can't speak my mind. I think they forget that we are actually ladies ourselves, and for them to be talking about cheating on their wife is not pleasant to hear. I would rather it wasn't spoken about at all – I don't need to hear it. If they need to speak with their wife, I would rather they left the room but sometimes they don't and sit winking at me. I have to smile sweetly and let them get on with it.

You might find that you end up having different views on some things. That's OK, but you need to be diplomatic and know when it's best to change the conversation to something positive and safe, like the weather!

Able to put your own personal problems and issues aside

Gentlemen book escorts for time out from their home and work life, so the last thing they want is to be burdened with your problems. Actually, I find my dates very therapeutic. Because I have to be focused on someone else, I can forget about my own troubles. I would never dream of turning up and moaning about my personal life, boyfriends, friends or work. Again, I hear horrible stories about girls breaking down and saying they are just doing it for the money; this puts the guy in a very awkward situation, and some girls purposefully do this and take advantage.

I know one escort that bragged to me that she had told a guy that she lived in a really dodgy part of Manchester (totally untrue) and that she feared for her safety, but couldn't afford to move anywhere else. He listened to her, advised her, didn't sleep with her because he felt guilty, and then ended up feeling so sorry for her that he helped her move to a safer, more expensive area *and* paid her mortgage! That is deceitful and totally inappropriate.

You must not talk about anything that implies you don't enjoy your job. If you don't enjoy it, don't do it! Once, I interviewed a lady to join an agency that I was thinking of setting up. She proceeded to tell me how she had three young boys by different fathers and that her house was threatened with repossession so she desperately needed the money. I knew she would say the same to any gentlemen she went to see!

A Good judge of character

I insist on speaking with potential dates on the phone – I don't mind contact by email initially, but I must speak to the gentleman to confirm a date. You have to go by your instincts. The people I enjoy meeting the most are those who seem to want to go out of their way to ensure my comfort. They ask if I have any preferences for hotels and food, and say they would like me to wear whatever I'm comfortable in. They don't ask about services, they are just happy to go with the flow. Sometimes I get it wrong, but generally I have been very lucky with the dates I've accepted, and I've had some wonderful experiences.

In addition to all of this, you must also:

Have a good sense of humour

Having a good sense of humour is a bonus. If you can make people laugh, you are on to a winner. Everybody likes to laugh. Men love cheeky, suggestive jokes.

Have a warm and friendly personality

If you are going to offer the 'Girlfriend Experience' then you need to have a warm and friendly personality because this will help put people at ease.

Not let anyone disrespect you

Being a GFE doesn't mean you have to put up with being treated with disrespect. If someone says or does the wrong thing, and it offends me, I let them know. After all, I'm a real person, with real feelings. If you feel uncomfortable about anything, it's OK to say so. Use your instincts, and don't let anyone treat you with anything other than respect. Gentlemen are paying for your time and company, but this does not entitle them to treat you badly. You are well within your rights to walk away. It depends on the situation and it's up to your discretion whether to return any of the gentleman's money.

People only disrespect you if you let them. At the end of the day, your health, safety and comfort are of paramount importance!

Glossary

Here is some of the sexual terminology used in the world of escorting...

69 Simultaneous fellatio and cunnilingus.
A Anal sex.
A-levels Anal sex.
AC/DC Bisexual (male or female).
AWO Anal sex without a condom.
Bareback Without a condom.
BBBJ Bareback Blow job – fellatio without a condom; not necessarily to completion.
BBBJTC Bareback blow job to completion.
BBF Bareback Fuck – sexual intercourse without a condom.
BBW Big Beautiful Woman.
BDSM Bondage and Discipline, Domination and Submission – sadomasochism.
BJ Blow job.
Breast Relief The man's penis is rubbed between a lady's breasts.

Brown Shower Defecation in a sexual context.

Butt Plug A small dildo used to stretch the anus, usually before anal sex.

Cappuccino After the man comes in the escort's mouth, she dribbles it out like a frothy coffee.

CIM Come In Mouth – the man ejaculates into the escort's mouth.

Clockwatcher Girl who leaves on the dot after her appointment has ended or sometimes before.

COB Come On Body. The man ejaculates over the escort's body.

COF Come On Face. The man ejaculates over the escort's face.

Completion Orgasm – OWO to completion means until you come.

Covered With a condom.

CP Corporal punishment.

Creampie Ejaculation in the vagina (or anus) without a condom.

Cunnilingus Oral sex on a woman.

Cut Man who is circumcised.

DATY Dining at the Y – oral sex on a woman.

DFK Deep French-kissing.

DP Double penetration – one penis in the vagina, another in the anus.

Extras Services charged extra for, such as anal sex or come in mouth.

Facial This is where the man ejaculates over the girl's face.

Fellatio Oral sex on a man.

Fisting A whole hand inserted into the vagina.

FS Full sex/service.

Full service Oral and vaginal sex.

Full strip Likely to mean that the lady takes all her clothes off.

GFE Girlfriend Experience.

Going down Oral sex.

GLOSSARY

Golden shower Urination in a sexual context. Usually means that the lady urinates over her client, or at least for the client to watch.

Greek Anal sex.

Half-strip Topless.

Hardsports *see* Brown Shower.

HJ Hand-job – the escort masturbates the client's penis.

Hobbyist US term for a regular user of an escort's services.

HR Hand-relief/hand-job.

HS Hardsports, *see* Brown Shower.

Incall The client visits the escort.

John Male client.

Massage parlour Officially offering massages, but extra services are usually offered separately.

MFF A male-female-female threesome.

MFS Massage and full service.

MILF Mother I'd Like To Fuck – a mature female escort.

Mish The missionary position.

MMF A male-male-female threesome.

O/O-levels Oral sex.

Outcall Where the escort visits the client in his home or hotel.

OW Oral with a condom.

OWO Oral without, *see* BBBJ.

OWOTC Oral without to completion.

Pearl necklace The man ejaculates over the girl's breasts/shoulders/neck.

Private Time Sexual services after dinner/theatre date.

Provider The service provider; i.e. the escort.

PSE Porn Star Experience.

Punter *see* John.

Raincoat Condom.

Reverse Client taking on a role that would usually be performed by an escort – for example, reverse oral is the client performing cunnilingus.

Rimming Anilingus.

Russian *see* Breast Relief.

Sandwich *see* DP.

Sausage Sandwich *see* Breast Relief.

Service Provider/SP *see* Provider.

SM or S&M Sado-masochism. *See also* BDSM.

Snowballing The guy ejaculates into a girl's mouth and they pass it between them, mouth to mouth.

Solid Sports *see* Brown Shower.

Stirring the porridge Vaginal sex after the girl has had unprotected sex.

Straight Sex Intercourse.

Submissive Lady who will allow the client to spank/cane her and generally submit to his will.

Swallows The escort swallows the client's semen.

Tit Fuck Breast Relief.

Toys Sex aids that the lady uses/inserts into herself such as dildos or vibrators.

Tromboning The escort kneels behind the man and rims him while giving a hand-job.

Uncovered Without a condom.

VFM Value for money.

Watersports/WS Urinating, either on someone or them on you.

www.miss-b.net